KETO DIET
CROCK
POT
Cookbook

First Published in 2018 by Amy Huckabee

ISBN-13: 978-1722660871
ISBN-10: 1722660872

Interior, Front and Back Cover Design by Amy Huckabee

Printed in the United States of America.

First Edition

Jolly Books Hub

CONTENTS

Lunch Recipes

Soup Recipes

Stew Recipes

Chili Recipes

Meat Recipes

Seafood Recipes

AUTHOR

"To my dearest Daniel"

A graduate of UCLA, Amy Huckabee M.D. earned her bachelor's degree in Health and Nutrition in 1992. She is a passionate advocate for the ketogenic diet and the health benefits it offers to millions of people worldwide. After a highly successful career helping millions of people lose weight, Amy has now retired gracefully to Los Angeles, CA. Every month Amy likes to give back to society by hosting ketogenic diet classes to help people lose weight in her local community. In her free time, Amy likes cooking, blogging, walking her two dogs Toby and Arthur and spending time with friends and family.

... Amy

Ketogenic 101

Keto 101

What is the Ketogenic Diet?

Unlike many other diets, this one is easy to understand! The ketogenic diet is simply a high fat, low carbohydrate diet that involves reducing your intake of carbs and replacing them with fats. When you eat foods that are high in carbs, your body produces two things: insulin and glucose.

- ✓ **Glucose** is a molecule needed by our bodies to convert and use the energy from the food we eat to fuel our body, typically carbohydrate.
- ✓ **Insulin** is a substance made by our pancreas to process glucose within our bloodstream.

Since glucose is our main source of energy, the fat we have stored away is therefore not needed and sits there unused. When deciding if the ketogenic diet is for them, many people choose a typical diet of eating foods high in carbs. We have been taught that carbs are needed for energy since we were tots. This is true, but only to a point.

Despite what you may have read, there are four types of ketogenic diet.

- ✓ High-Protein Ketogenic Diet: This type of keto diet involves eating lots of protein. The ratio required to stick to this type of diet is 60% fat, 35% protein and 5% carbohydrates.

✓ Targeted Ketogenic Diet (Tkd): If you like the freedom of having some room to move around on a diet, this one is for you! You can intake more carbs if you are working out as well.

✓ Cyclical Ketogenic Diet (Ckd): This type requires periods of high-carb intake—for example, 5 ketogenic days paired with a few high-carb consumption days.

✓ Standard Ketogenic Diet (Skd): This type of keto diet is the most popular and recommended. It requires you to consume moderate amounts of protein and high amounts of fat. It is based around this popular macro: 75% fat, 20% protein and 5% carbs.

The standard ketogenic diet is the most popular diet for beginners, but you may find that the other three diets are better suited to your body and personal goals. For now, however, I suggest that you start with the standard ketogenic diet to see how your body adapts and to minimize any side affects you may experience on the diet. Many of my students also start with the standard diet and their weight loss results have been excellent because they have exceeded my expectations every time.

History of the Ketogenic Diet

The ketogenic diet has a long and rich history, predating most of the diet trends and fads on the market today. Beginning in the 1920s and 1930s, an early form of the ketogenic diet was used to treat patients with epilepsy. This was the only help patients had until medications were developed in later years—for example, insulin injections. An interesting fact is that in 20% to 30% of all cases, the ketogenic diet remains more effective than medications in treating epilepsy. Today, despite our medical advancements, the ketogenic diet is still used by practitioners as an alternative remedy for treating epilepsy.

In slightly more technical terms, in 1921, an endocrinologist by the name of Rollin Woodyatt, discovered that the ketogenic diet enables our liver to produce three water-soluble compounds. These are:

- ✓ β-hydroxybutyrate
- ✓ acetoacetate
- ✓ acetone

Together, these compounds are known as ketone bodies. During the early 20th Century, an American by the name of Bernarr Macfadden introduced fasting as a means of improving health and wellbeing. His student osteopath, Hugh Conklin, then introduced fasting as a treatment to control epilepsy. Coklin proposed that epileptic seizures are caused by a toxin secreted in the intestine and suggested that fasting for 18 to 25 days could cause the toxin to disappear completely. His epileptic patients were put on a 'water diet', which he reported cured both children and adults with the condition. An analysis of the study performed showed that 20% of Coklin's patients became seizure-free, while 50% demonstrated remarkable improvement. Fasting therapy was soon adopted as part of mainstream therapy for epilepsy and in 1916, Dr McMurray reported to the New York Medical Journal that he had successfully treated epileptic patients by prescribing fasting, followed by a diet free of starch and sugar.

Moving on to the 1960s, Russel Wilder, a medical student, coined the phrase 'ketogenic diet' for its official use in the treatment of epilepsy. After considerable research in the 1960s, scientists found that medium-chain triglycerides produced even more ketones per unit of energy. This led to a revised ketogenic diet for epilepsy patients formulated by Peter Huttenlocher. Here, 60 percent of a patient's daily calorie intake now came in the form of MCT oil. Accordingly, a larger variety of meals were now available for sufferers, and so the ketogenic diet was born.

Ultimately, this was a significant discovery because it meant that patients could eat more carbohydrates and proteins, which lead to the possibility of a varied diet. And now we have the history behind the diet, let's look at it more **closely**.

Science of the Ketogenic Diet

Ketosis

The most important point to understand is that the ketogenic diet is a low carbohydrate, high fat diet. The intention behind it is for your body to produce ketones as a source of energy. This happens when your body transitions into a state called ketosis. This is achieved by eating fewer carbs (5% to 10%), more fat (60% to 75%) and moderate protein (15% to 30%).

Normally, your bodies process the carbohydrate we eat on an average balanced diet by turning it into glucose for energy. When ketosis is reached, your body begins to use the ketones produced from the transfer of fat to energy. If ketosis is maintained, your body can enter a metabolic state where it will continue to burn these ketones. Ketosis is not a foreign process for your body. It happens naturally when your glucose levels are lowThis process also helps improve your body's resistance to insulin and is an excellent choice for diabetics. We mentioned ketones, but what exactly are they? When our body breaks down fat for energy, certain byproducts are produced. These are known as ketone bodies or ketones for short. This process works as follows:

- ✓ When your body doesn't have enough glucose, your glycogen levels eventually run out.
- ✓ Your body now begins to burn fuel differently since the glycogen stores have now depleted. It does this by using fat to fuel itself.
- ✓ Your liver will start to produce ketones that fuel your body.
- ✓ When your body reaches this state, you are now under ketosis.

This process produces three ketone bodies we discussed earlier on:

- ✓ β-hydroxybutyrate
- ✓ acetoacetate
- ✓ acetone

Your metabolism is happy burning carbohydrates for fuel. Simple sugars from bread, rice and candy are broken down with little thought or energy, providing you with enough fuel to get through the day. When provided steady sources of carbohydrate throughout the day, things run smoothly. The problem is, unless you are giving your body only what it needs for carbohydrates, the rest of those simple sugars will be stored as fat to use later, perhaps if you miss a meal. Weight gain happens when you consistently eat more than your body needs to survive. Physiologically speaking, this is necessary, so you don't keel over between meals, but these days, inactivity plus huge portions mean you will keep storing fuel you don't intend to burn—you gain weight.

When you do not have a source of steady carbohydrates during the day, your metabolism shifts to pull fat from your stores, and burn it for energy. This fat-burning process is called ketosis, and the byproduct of this is ketones. Ketosis is the body's natural back up to burning carbohydrates as a matter of survival. As you could imagine, ketosis helps you lose weight because you are constantly burning fat for fuel instead of burning carbs as they come into your system. The problem is, it takes a bit of time to enter ketosis, and as soon as you eat carbohydrates, your body goes back to burning sugars. The good news is that you can build your diets around proteins and fats instead of carbohydrates to mimic carbohydrate starvation to push your body into ketosis.

While everyone will be a little bit different, the threshold of carbohydrates is about 50–60 grams per day, and about 10–15 grams per meal, before you exit ketosis. To put this into perspective, 15 grams is equal to a small slice of bread, which is not allowed on the ketogenic diet. To make the most of meals, most of these carbs will be in sources like vegetables with low carb content. The basic ketogenic meal is a combination of proteins like chicken and fish, with a large side of non-starchy vegetables like salad and zucchini. Fats can be used without real restriction too, so healthy fats like olive oil and avocado can be used to make up for the calories not taken up by carbohydrate-rich starches like rice and potato.

The primary goal of maintaining ketosis on the ketogenic diet is to force your body into a metabolic state. You do not want to do this through starvation, but rather through the starvation of carbohydrates. Our bodies are very adaptable, so when you switch your diet by loading it with fats instead of carbs, you burn ketones as an energy source. When you get to burning off optimal ketone levels, you then can lose weight faster and experience the physical and mental performance benefits the ketogenic diet has to offer.

The Process of Ketosis

A form of acidosis, ketosis disrupts the pH balance in your body due to the presence of more ketones in the blood. Ketones are a byproduct of your fat metabolism that are released when fat is broken down into an energy source. Metabolism on ketosis is when blood sugars are not readily available to your body as a source of energy, your body switches gears and starts to break down fat instead. When the ketones are broken down into glucose and released into your bloodstream, this is the start of ketosis. Produced in the liver, ketones can be utilized for other metabolic processes in your body. Getting to the point that you reach ketosis may seem complicated to those that are new to the keto diet. But overall, it is a straightforward process:

- ✓ Restrict carbs: Many people focus only on their intake of net carbs when they should be limiting total carbs. Try your best to stay below 20g of net carbs and 35g of total carbs.
- ✓ Restrict protein consumption: There are many folks who switch to the ketogenic diet from other diets and totally space off limiting their intake of protein. Eating too much protein can lead to drastically low levels of ketones, limiting ketosis. For sustained weight loss, you want to eat around 0.6–0.8 grams per pound to achieve that lean body mass you desire.
- ✓ Don't fret over fat: Fat is the primary source of energy on the keto diet, so you need to make it a priority to fuel your body with enough of it. Despite popular

belief, you are going to lose less weight if you starve yourself, no matter what diet you are on, so avoid this always.

✓ Drink water: When you first begin the keto diet, make it a goal to drink a gallon of water per day. This sounds like a lot, but you must stay hydrated to regulate your bodily functions and control your levels of hunger.

✓ Quit with the snacks: You can lose weight much easier when your body doesn't undergo multiple spikes in insulin throughout the day. Snacking for no reason can stall your weight loss achievements.

✓ Fast: Fasting is a good tool to help boost your ketone levels.

  o Skip a meal: Skipping a meal induces fasting. You can decide what meal to skip.

  o Limit your intake of food to a 4–7 hours window and leave the remaining time to fast.

  o 24–48-hour cleanses are when you do not eat for 1–2 days and experience extended fasting periods.

✓ Incorporate exercise: Exercise is a healthy habit for everyone. If you want to get the most out of undergoing the ketogenic diet, add 20-30 minutes to your regular exercise routine each day. Even an extra walk can help regulate blood sugar and promote more weight loss.

✓ Begin supplementing: This is not always needed, but it can help you get the best out of the keto diet.

There are several resources that you will come across in your hunt for achieving optimal ketosis. I recommend putting all those articles to the side because the most effective ketosis can be achieved easily through diet and nutrition. There is no magic pill, shortcut, or gimmick that will ultimately help you accomplish it. There is one method of measuring your ketosis levels that involves you urinating on a strip of paper, but these can be inaccurate and can cost a lot of money. Instead, know the physical symptoms that will naturally tell you that you are on the right track:

- ✓ Increased urination: The keto diet is a natural diuretic that increases acetoacetate, a ketone body that is excreted through the process of urinating.
- ✓ Dry mouth: Thanks to having to urinate more often, this can lead to dry mouth and being thirsty. This is another reason to drink lots of water so that you replenish your electrolytes effectively.
- ✓ Bad breath: A ketone body known as acetone is excreted into our mouth which affects the smell of our breath. It tends to smell like ripe fruit, sometimes even as potent as nail polish remover. This is temporary and goes away over time.
- ✓ Reduced hunger and increased energy: After you get past the "keto flu" stage, you will experience higher energy levels, a clear state of mind and will be hungry less often.
- ✓ Keto flu: This type of flu is a common phenomenon for newbies on the ketogenic diet, but thankfully it goes away after just a few days. You might experience mild discomfort in the form of cramps, nausea, headaches and fatigue.
- ✓ The following food wheel gives you an idea of the five main food groups and should serve as a helpful starting point for selecting the right foods for ketosis.

Ketoacidosis

There is often a lot of confusion when it comes to the difference between ketosis and ketoacidosis. Ketoacidosis happens in individuals who are diabetic and is often a complication of type 1 diabetics. It results from high levels of ketones in blood sugars, which can be life-threatening. This can make the blood too acidic, which has the potential to change the overall function of vital internal organs. This is not to be confused with the process of ketosis on the ketogenic diet.

Know Your Macros!

Macros is the abbreviation for the term macronutrients or the "big 3", comprising carbohydrates, protein and fats. You can use the macro calculator for figuring out what your personal daily needs should be. Fats are 10% anti-ketogenic and 90% ketogenic, thanks to the tiny bit of glucose that is released as our bodies convert the triglycerides. Proteins are 58% anti-ketogenic and 45% ketogenic because insulin levels are risen from half of the proteins we ingest that are converted to glucose. Carbs are 100% anti-ketogenic since they are responsible for the rise in insulin and blood glucose levels. What does this mean? Simply that carbs and protein hurt the act of trying to get into the state of ketosis. So, it is vital to learn how they are being converted to energy, which is through metabolic pathways after being ingested as nutrients.

Your Body on the Ketogenic Diet

With all this new information, you may be wondering how you will physically be feeling when you first start undergoing the keto transformation. Your body is more than likely accustomed to a simple routine of breaking down the carbohydrates you consume into energy. Your body has already built up the enzymes it needs to process these carbs, which means they are by no means used to dealing with the breaking down and storage of fats. This means that your body is having to deal with and become used to a lack of glucose but an increase in fat consumption, which means it must produce a whole new supply of enzymes. Once your body starts to become used to the state of ketosis, you will naturally shift to utilize what glucose you have left in storage. Therefore, your muscles will have a depleted supply of glycogen, which can mean lethargy and a lack of overall energy.

During the first week of undergoing the keto diet, many people report being dizzy, easily aggravated and headaches. This is because your electrolytes are flushed from your system. Another reason is to drink lots of water and keep up with your sodium intake: salt helps you to retain water, which replenishes your electrolytes.

Side Effects of the Ketogenic Diet

The keto flu

This type of flu is a common phenomenon for newbies on the ketogenic diet, but thankfully it goes away just after a few days. You might also experience mild discomfort in the form of cramps, nausea, headaches and fatigue.

The keto flu occurs due to two main reasons:

1. You are going to the bathroom more often to urinate, which means you are losing electrolytes and water within the body. You can combat this easily by drinking a bouillon cube in water.

2. Your body is in a phase of total transition. You are used to processing a higher intake of carbohydrates. Your body needs a bit of time to create the enzymes needed to process a higher intake of fat. Therefore, you may feel low on energy. It is best to gradually decrease your intake of carbs and not go cold turkey.

Once you increase your water consumption and replace electrolytes, you will find that the symptoms of the keto flu decrease or totally diminish. For a person that is beginning the transition to the ketogenic diet, it is recommended to eat less than 15 grams of carbs a day and decrease this amount over time. All good things in life tend to have a bad side. Luckily, these risks are not near as negative as ones you have the chance to experience on other diets.

✓ **Fatigue and irritability** – Even though raised ketone levels can drastically improve a few areas regarding your physical quality of life, they are also directly related to feeling tired and having to work harder during physical activities.

✓ **"Brain fog"** – If you stay on the ketogenic diet long term, there is going to be a major shifting when it comes to the metabolic areas of your body. This can make you moody and somewhat sluggish, which can make you not able to think clearly or adequately focus. Ensure that you are reducing your levels of carb intake at steady levels, not all at once.

✓ **Lipids may change** – Even though fats on the ketogenic diet are welcomed, if you consume large amounts of saturated fats, your cholesterol levels will begin to increase. Make sure you are consuming healthy fats.

✓ **Micronutrient deficiencies** – Diets that consist of low-carb foods are more than likely lacking in essential nutrients, such as magnesium, potassium and iron. You might want to strongly consider finding a high-quality multivitamin to take daily.

✓ **Developing ketoacidosis** – If your ketone levels become too out of whack, it may lead to this condition. pH levels within your blood decrease, creating an environment that is high in acidity, which can be threatening for those with diabetes.

✓ **Muscle loss** – As you consume less energy, your body leans on the help of other tissues as a source of fuel. If you work out heavily while on a diet like the ketogenic diet, there is the potential for major muscle loss.

Benefits of the Ketogenic Diet

All types of low-carb diets have been on the table of controversy for quite a few years. It has been said that diets high in fat content can raise cholesterol levels through the roof, causing heart disease and other bad body ailments. But research has shown that amongst other diets, low-carb ones win the race. They are not only a great substitute when trying to lose weight, but they even have other great health benefits, even reducing cholesterol levels. Here are some ways that the Ketogenic Diet can produce some good things in your life!

The main component that is largely working in your body during your time on the ketogenic diet is the process of ketosis. Creating this metabolic state has been proven to have drastically positive effects, even if only on the diet for a short time. Here are some grand benefits of ketosis itself first!

- ✓ Increases our body's capabilities to use fats as a source of fuel.
- ✓ Ketosis has a protein-sparing effect, which means our bodies prefer utilizing ketones as opposed to glucose.
- ✓ Lowers levels of insulin within our bodies, which contains a lipolysis-blocking effect, which reduces the utilization of fatty acids as a source of energy. When insulin levels are lowered, growth hormones and other growth factors can then be released without an issue.
- ✓ Suppresses hunger – Naturally, many diets require you to eat less than your body is used to. Because of this, never-ending hunger pains always seem to strike and at the worst times. This is the main reason people tend to feel miserable while on any diet plan. Diets that are low in carb intake are great because it automatically reduces your appetite. Those who cut carbs and consume more proteins and fat actually eat *fewer* calories.
- ✓ More potential for weight loss – People who stick within the means of low-carb diets lose weight at a much faster rate than those who within the means of a low-carb diet. Diets low in carbohydrates tend to help in the reduction of excess water in our bodies, which can add on the pounds. The ketogenic diet reduces insulin levels too, meaning the kidneys are shedding excess sodium that can lead to retaining extra weight.
- ✓ Reduction of triglycerides – This is a fancy name for fat molecules. These little boogers contribute to ailments such as heart disease. When people reduce the consumption of carbs, there is quite a lessening of triglycerides building up in our bodies.

✓ Increase of good cholesterol levels – HDL is the kind of cholesterol you *want* to have. The ketogenic diet helps with raising HDL levels because of the consumption of fats. There are major bodily improvements when the levels of good and bad cholesterol start to shift.

✓ Reduces blood sugar and insulin levels – When we consume carbs, they are broken into simple sugars by our digestive system. They then go into our bloodstreams and elevate blood sugar levels. High sugars can be toxic, which is why insulin exists. There are many people who have a type of diabetes not only because of bloodlines and genetics, but because they have not eaten the best for quite a bit of their life. Their bodies no longer recognize insulin when it is attempting to help lower blood sugar levels. With the ketogenic diet, it has been seen that blood sugar and insulin levels come way down.

✓ Reduction in blood pressure – Diets that are low in carbohydrates are effective in reducing blood pressure levels, which can assist us in living longer. When blood pressure is high, we are at greater risks of developing hypertension and other ailments.

✓ Natural treatment for cancer – Properly regulating your body's metabolic functions has been proven to be a great step in reducing and even treating cancer. Reducing or totally removing carbs from your diet can help in the deletion of energy from cancerous cells and stop them from spreading.

✓ Effective in treating metabolic syndrome – This syndrome is actually a serious medical condition that is associated with heart disease and diabetes. There are several symptoms:

   ✓ Low levels of HDL
   ✓ High triglyceride levels
   ✓ Raised fasting blood sugar levels
   ✓ Elevated blood pressure
   ✓ Abdominal obesity

✓ Therapy for some brain disorders – There are certain areas of our brains that strictly run on glucose as a fuel. This is the reason behind why our livers produce it from protein if we do not consume carbs. There are bigger portions of our brains, however, that burn through ketones. Think back to Charlie Abraham, who was mentioned earlier in this chapter. In studies, more than half of children who utilized the ketogenic diet had a 50% reduction in seizures.

Foods to Avoid

✓ Grains: Rice, corn, oats, wheat, barley, etc. Pasta, bread, cookies, crackers, etc.

✓ Factory-farmed fish and pork

✓ Processed foods

✓ Artificial sweeteners

✓ Refined fats and oils

✓ Foods that are "low-fat," "low-carb" or "zero-carb"

✓ Milk

✓ Alcoholic and sweet beverages

✓ Soy products

Foods to Eat

Any diet can be challenging when you are not aware of what to eat and what not to eat. Thankfully, you have an entire list of ketogenic must and must-not eats to ensure you stay on the right track!

Grass-Fed and Wild Animal Sources	Healthy Fats	Non-Starchy veggies	Fruits	Beverages and Condiments
Beef	**Saturated**	**Leafy greens**	Avocado	Water
Lamb				Black coffee
Goat	Coconut oil	Radicchio	**Berries** mulberries	Tea
Venison	Butter	Endive	cranberries	Pork rinds
Fish and seafood	Ghee	Chives	raspberries	Mayo
Pork	Goose fat	Chard	strawberries	Mustard
Poultry	Duck fat	Lettuce	blueberries	Pesto
Eggs	Chicken fat	Spinach	blackberries	Bone Broth
Gelatin	Tallow	Bok choy		Pickles and other
Ghee	Lard	Swiss chard	Sugar snap peas	fermented eats
Liver, heart,			Artichokes	Spices
kidneys, and	**Monounsaturated**	**Cruciferous**	Water chestnuts	Lemon/lime juice &
other organ		**vegetables**	Sea vegetables	zest
meats	Olive oil			Whey protein
	Macadamia oil	Radishes	**Root veggies**	
Nuts & Seeds	Avocado oil	Kohlrabi	pumpkin	
Sunflower seeds		Dark leaf kale	winter squash	
Pecans	**Polyunsaturated**	Celery	mushrooms	
Almonds		Asparagus	Cabbage	
Walnuts	Fatty fish and seafood	Cucumber	Cauliflower	
Hazelnuts		Summer squash	Broccoli	
Macadamia nuts		(spaghetti squash,	Fennel	
		zucchini)	Brussels sprouts	
		Bamboo shoots		

Understanding Fats

Since fats make up a large and important portion of your keto diet, they are vital for staying healthy and in shape. But it is not just consuming fat this is crucial, but choosing the right fats is important as well! There can be a lot of confusion as to what fats are good, bad, and those which should be avoided when cooking with your Instant Pot. Here we will break down those good and bad fats.

Good Fats

The "good guy" fats that are a go in your diet are split up into four different categories:

1. Saturated Fats
2. Monounsaturated fats (MUFAs)
3. Polyunsaturated fats (PUFAs)
4. Trans fats (naturally occurring)

When it boils down to "what types of aspects are in what fats," you must remember that all fats in the world are created by a mixture of all the above types of fat but are categorized by which one is the most dominant. Here, we will break down each type of fat when it comes to consuming foods with your Instant Pot. This will help you to easily see them when you are making decisions about what to fuel your body and mind with.

Saturated Fats

These fats had a bad reputation for many years. They were viewed as terrible for the health of your heart and we were taught to avoid them.

However, since then there have been various studies that prove this wrong by showing no significant link between saturated fats and the risk of heart disease. We have been consuming saturated fats for *thousands* of years. Considering this new information, there is a plethora of great benefits that come along with the inclusion of healthy saturated fats in your daily diet.

Several saturated fats include something we call "medium-chain triglycerides (MCTs)," which are found in items like coconut oil and small amounts of butter and palm oil. MCT can be digested simply and easily in the body. When we eat these MCT's, they pass through the liver and are utilized automatically as an energy source! This means they are superb in your diet if you want to lose weight or boost your physical performance.

Health benefits of saturated fats:

- ✓ Increase in the function of the immune system
- ✓ Better cholesterol levels, both HDL and LDL
- ✓ Better HDL to LDL cholesterol ratio
- ✓ Improved maintenance of bone density
- ✓ Rise of HDL (good) cholesterol to prevent LDL within the arteries
- ✓ Promotes the creation of hormones like cortisol and testosterone, which are important for various reasons

Best sources of saturated fats:

- ✓ Butter
- ✓ Cocoa butter
- ✓ Coconut oil
- ✓ Cream
- ✓ Eggs
- ✓ Lard
- ✓ Palm oil
- ✓ Red meat

Monounsaturated Fats

Unlike saturated fats, monounsaturated fatty acids (MUFAs) have been a graciously accepted "good fat" for a long time. There have been a variety of studies that have directly linked MUFA's with benefits such as insulin resistance and good cholesterol levels.

Health benefits of MUFAs:

- ✓ Better levels of HDL cholesterol
- ✓ Decrease in blood pressure
- ✓ Decreased risk of developing heart disease
- ✓ Decrease in belly fat
- ✓ Decrease in insulin resistance

Best sources of MUFAs to eat:

- ✓ Avocados and avocado oil
- ✓ Extra virgin olive oil
- ✓ Goose fat
- ✓ Lard and bacon fat
- ✓ Macadamia nut oil

Polyunsaturated Fats

When it comes to consuming polyunsaturated fatty acids (PUFAs), it boils most importantly down to the type. When PUFAs are heated up, they can create free radicals, which are harmful to the body and responsible in the increase of inflammation and have been shown to increase the risk of developing cancer and heart disease. In other words, the majority of PUFAs should be eaten in cold forms and should never be utilized for cooking.

PUFAs can be found in processed oils and other extremely healthy sources. Eating the correct kinds of PUFAs can give you benefits, especially when you incorporate them into your diet. They include Omega 3's and Omega 6's, which are essential to feeling great!

The amount of PUFA's that you eat is extremely crucial. The ratio of omega 3 to omega 6 should be around 1:1. But most of Western diets consume a ratio of 1:30.

Health benefits of PUFAs:

When you consume a good balance of omega 3 and omega 6, you greatly reduce the risk of developing the following:

- ✓ Autoimmune disorders and other inflammatory diseases
- ✓ Heart disease
- ✓ Intake of PUFAs may even help improve symptoms of depression and help those with ADHD, which are more benefits associated with a keto diet.
- ✓ Stroke

Best sources of PUFA's to eat:

- ✓ Avocado oil
- ✓ Chia seeds
- ✓ Extra virgin olive oil
- ✓ Fatty fish and fish oil
- ✓ Flaxseeds and flaxseed oil
- ✓ Nut oils
- ✓ Sesame oil
- ✓ Walnuts

Trans Fats

You are probably questioning the author's intelligence seeing trans fats under the "good" fats category. But it does have a right to be in this section! Yes, the majority of trans fats are wildly unhealthy and can be very harmful to the human body, there *is* a type of trans fat, known as *vaccenic acid*, that is good for you! It is naturally found in foods like grass-fed meats and dairy products.

Health benefits of vaccenic acid can include:

- ✓ Decreased risk of developing diabetes and obesity
- ✓ Decreased risk of developing heart disease
- ✓ Protection against developing cancer

Best sources of healthy and natural trans fats to eat:

- ✓ Dairy fats such as butter and yogurt
- ✓ Grass-fed animal products

Bad Fats

One of the positive aspects that attract many people to the keto diet is that they can consume lots of satisfying foods and healthy fats. But, lurking around the corner, there are also bad fats that you must keep an eye on. You want to get rid of and eliminate these pesky guys, so you don't damage your bodily health. One of the key things to remember is that the quality of the food genuinely matters.

Processed Trans and Polyunsaturated Fats

Processed trans fats are a common type of fat that many of you are familiar with. They have the capability of being wildly detrimental to your overall physical wellbeing.

Artificial trans fats are created during the production of food, which occurs when polyunsaturated fats are processed. Therefore, it's important to only choose PUFAs that are unprocessed that are not overheated or altered in any way. Not The processing of PUFAs creates free radicals that are harmful when consumed and they are made from oils that contain genetically modified seeds.

Risks of consuming trans fats include:
- ✓ Bad for the health of your gut
- ✓ Increased risk of developing cancer
- ✓ Increased risk of developing heart disease
- ✓ Lead cause of inflammatory health issues
- ✓ Decrease in the good HDL cholesterol and increase of bad LDL cholesterol

Examples of trans fats to *eliminate*:
- ✓ Hydrogenated and partially hydrogenated oils that are in processed products like cookies, crackers, margarine, and fast food
- ✓ Processed vegetable oils like cottonseed, sunflower, safflower, soybean, and canola oils

Steps to Success on the Ketogenic Diet

This chapter is full of fool-proof ways to keep yourself on track as your venture down the Instant Pot road.

✓ **Hydration**: This should be something you do daily already but consume 32 ounces of water within the first hour that you get out of bed in the morning and strive to drink up another 32-48 ounces before the noon hour. Drink at *least* half of your weight in ounces of water or close to your full body weight in ounces daily to keep your overall hydration at healthy levels.

✓ **Practice intermittent fasting**: Start reducing your carb intake a couple to a few days before getting down and dirty. Break your day down into two phases:

- o **Building phase:** Amount of time between first and last meal
- o **Cleaning phase:** Amount of time between last and first meal

Start with a 12-16-hour cleaning phase and an 8-12-hour building phase. Your body will adapt over time, which will enable you to move to a 4-6-hour building time paired with an 18-20-hour cleaning phase each day.

Eat lots of salt: We are reminded all the time to lower our consumption of sodium. When you undergo a low-carb diet, insulin levels decrease, and our kidneys excrete higher levels of sodium. This results in a lowering of our sodium/potassium ratio.

- o Add ¼ teaspoon of pink salt to glasses of water
- o Add kelp, nori or dulse to dishes
- o Be generous with amount of pink salt you add to food
- o Consume pumpkin seeds or macadamia nuts as a snack
- o Drink organic broth off and on throughout the day
- o Eat cucumber or celery; both have natural sodium

✓ Exercise on a regular basis: High-intensity exercise daily help to assist in activating glucose molecules known as GLUT-4 which are responsible for reciting information to various areas of the body back to the liver and muscle tissues. This receptor takes away sugar that is in the bloodstream and uses it as muscle and liver glycogen. Exercising on a regular basis doubles the levels of crucial proteins in both the muscles and liver.

✓ Work on improving mobility of bowels: Many people struggle with constipation issues. To help, consume fermented edibles, such as sauerkraut, coconut water, kimchi, etc. It is recommended to take extra supplements, such as magnesium. Drinking one green drink per day will also help to increase the levels of calcium, magnesium, and potassium in your system, all of which help aid constipation and promote healthy bowel movement.

✓ Don't eat too much protein: Even though consumption of proteins is recommended following a keto diet, some people do not know a proper balance and eat too much protein. Your body will change all those amino acids into glucose through the process known as gluconeogenesis if you eat too much protein. You will probably have to play with the amounts of protein you eat because some people need than others.

✓ Choose your carbs wisely: For a keto diet, it is best to consume at least some good types of carbohydrates, such as starchy veggies and fruits likes berries, apples or citrus. Combine them into a green smoothie for a great morning pick-me-up!

✓ Utilize mct oil: The usage of high-quality medium chain triglyceride (MCT) is crucial for replenishing your energy levels throughout the day. You can cook with this oil as well as add it to coffee, tea, green drinks, protein shakes and more!

✓ Keep stress to a minimum: The buildup of daily stress will inhibit our energy levels. If you are under constant chronic stress, then now may not be the time to undergo any form of diet, but rather a diet that concentrates on being anti-inflammatory and lower in carbs instead.

✓ Improve the quality of sleep: If you are not getting adequate amounts of rest, this is another aspect that can lead to a rise in stress hormones. Ensure that you are in a dark room that you feel comfortable in. It is recommended to get around 7-9 hours of sleep per night. The more stressed you are, the more sleep you need. Ensure that you are sleeping in a room that is no warmer than 65-70 degrees.

✓ Consume Ghee: Ghee is a great substitute for butter, if not a total replacement! It is highly recommended, and you can use it as normally as you utilize butter.

✓ Take omega-3's: It is important to consume or take Omega-3 vitamins. You should have higher levels of Omega 3's than Omega 6's in your diet. Eating all that oil will cause you harm if your Omega's are not properly balanced.

✓ Avoid alcohol: While this sounds like a bummer, the consumption of alcohol can put a stop to your weight loss. Which is worth it: that bottle of beer or being able to fit into those clothes you are hanging on to in hopes you will once again fit into them?

✓ Make lemon water your best friend: Not only is it tasty and refreshing, but lemon water helps to balance out your pH levels, which can create the perfect environment.

✓ Avoid "sugar-free" products: Even though it sounds better for you, try to avoid products that say "sugar-free" or "light" because these more than likely have more carbs than their original counterparts.

✓ Avoid low-fat: You should steer clear and not waste your precious time with anything that is low in fat. You need to have high percentages of fat in your diet in order to maintain an adequate and healthy balance. Otherwise, the protein you consume may be converted into sugars too.

✓ Get a food scale: This tool is important to have in your kitchen if you want total success. Being accurate is vital to the process of monitoring what you are fueling your body with. If you plan to track carbs and count calories, you really need to know what you are consuming. Make sure the scale you buy has a conversion button, an automatic shutoff, a tare function, as well as a removable plate.

✓ Know healthy alternatives to carbs: You will inevitably have cravings from time to time. There is something about fried chicken, rice, sauces, and more that make your mouth water. For ultimate satisfaction, it is a good idea to have alternatives and substitutes up your sleeve to combat. Try some of these alternatives!

- **Shirataki noodles** are low-carb, which makes them a perfect alternative when you have a hankering for pasta!

- **Cauliflower rice** can be used in the place of regular white or brown rice.

- **Spaghetti squash** can be creatively turned into noodles with the help of a spiralizer or simply with a fork. Awesome taste and less than half the carbs and calories.

- Use **heavy whipping cream** or **almond milk** in your coffee instead of that calorie-packed creamer.

- For those that love and constantly crave bread, there are many low-carb options, such as **low-carb bread and tortillas**!

- You will find that when your sweet tooth needs a bit of love that making shakes or smoothies with the help of **protein powder.** There are tons of flavors that can be easily mixed into batters, snacks, and much more! Plus, it gives you a nice boost of protein without sacrificing all the hard work you have put into eating a keto diet.

Crock Pot 101

What is a Crock Pot?

We rely on them for our soups, stews and easy weeknight dinners. They help make tough meat more tender and can even be used to make bread. We also toss around their names interchangeably, thinking that Crock Pots and slow cookers are interchangeable names for the same thing.

A Crock-Pot is a slow cooker. The Crock-Pot was first introduced in 1970 and was originally marketed as a bean cooker. Over time it was redesigned, and eventually evolved into the model we recognize today. Many companies now make crockpot-style slow cookers, and they are of course in wide use throughout the country.

Crock-Pots and slow cookers use moist heat to cook food over a long period of time. Both are used to cook the same types of foods, and both produce the same delicious results. These wonderful, small kitchen appliances even contain the same three components: a pot, glass lid and heating element. A crockpot is a brand of slow cooker that gave rise to a type of slow cooker. But a slow cooker is not always a crockpot!

This small electric appliance, a staple of many homes for more than 30 years, is based on the principle of slow cooking. The concept of slow cooking is simple: put food into some sort of container or contained area and let it cook slowly. It's a method used in barbecue pits and pig roasts, where low temperatures and a lot of time allow meat to become tender. Slow cooking can be done via dry heat, as in an oven or roaster, or it can be moist, by involving liquid during the cooking process. Slow cookers use moisture in a unique way because they remain sealed during the cooking process. As food cooks and lets off steam, the condensation collects inside.

The slow cooking method has been around for centuries, and the electrical slow cooker first became popular in the 1970s kitchen -- the original slow cookers came in chic colors of the day, such as avocado and goldenrod. But when microwaves came into vogue a few years later, the slow cooker was left behind as people started zapping their food. However, the tide has turned back to slow cooking and new cookbooks that provide a variety of tasty recipes for this one-pot wonder. Manufacturers developed newer, more stylish versions of the device, which led to its resurgence over the last decade as a must-have appliance for time-strapped cooks. In the next section, we'll look at how a pot for preparing beans revolutionized cooking.

Cooking with the Crock Pot

The slow cooker was developed from an electrical bean pot, a pot that was invented in the 1960s to steep dry beans. A slow cooker has three main components: an outer casing, an inner container and a lid

The outer casing is metal and contains low-wattage heating coils, the component responsible for cooking the food, and these heating coils are completely encapsulated by the outer casing. The inner container, which is also called a crock, is made of glazed ceramic and fits inside the metal heating element. In some models, you can remove this cooking crock from the outer shell. The third piece of the appliance is a domed lid that fits tightly onto the crock.

The appliance cooks based on a combination of wattage and time. When turned on, the electrical coils heat up and transfer heat indirectly from the outer casing to the space between the base wall and the stoneware container. This indirect heat warms the crock to between 180 and 300 degrees Fahrenheit (82 to 149 degrees Celsius). This method of heat transfer simmers the ingredients inside the crock at a low temperature for several hours, until the food is thoroughly cooked.

As the food cooks, it releases steam, which the lid traps. The condensation creates a vacuum seal between the lid and the rim of the crock, which adds moisture to the food while helping the cooking process -- the lid is integral to the cooking process. The slow cooker typically has three settings: low, high and off. In programmable slow cookers, the device will switch to a warm setting after it has cooked the food to keep the meal at a proper temperature.

Cooking the Right Foods

The crockpot is a highly versatile appliance that can cook a variety of foods. Meats are one of the most popular items to cook in a crockpot, but they need to be thawed beforehand or they'll take too long to cook. When cooking meat, it's important to heat the meat to 140 degrees Fahrenheit (60 degrees Celsius) as quickly as possible to kill any bacteria. Always make sure the internal temperature of the meat is within recommended guidelines before serving. When cooking poultry, use poultry with the skin still attached because this will help keep the meat moist throughout the cooking process. Prepping vegetables for slow cooking may take longer to prepare than the meat and it's important to cut them uniformly so they'll cook evenly. Vegetables may also take longer to cook than meat, so when preparing stews or meat-and-vegetable dishes, layer the vegetables on the bottom of the pot.

Some of the best crockpot meals are soups and stews because the crockpot is designed to simmer on the low setting for long periods of time. Cover soup ingredients with water, and if you need to add more liquid during cooking, bring it to a boil first, so it doesn't lower the soup's cooking temperature. Dips and spreads are another category where crockpots shine. The low heat keeps a cheese-based dip warm without burning the ingredients and maintaining a dip at a low heat prevents ingredients from congealing during a party.

Grains are sometimes a surprising way to use a slow cooker. Oatmeal, cracked wheat and rice porridge can be cooked to provide a hot, nutritious breakfast.

Bread and bread-based dishes like stuffing can also be baked in a slow cooker—the low heat setting also helps bread dough rise. Another surprising slow-cooking category is desserts. While rice and tapioca puddings may seem like a no-brainer, you can also use slow cookers to make hot fruit desserts and even cakes.

Some recipes call for adding ingredients near the end of the cooking time because of the nature of the ingredients and their tolerance for the slow-cooking process. Spices and herbs may become too concentrated during cooking, so be sure to adjust their levels at the end of the process. Likewise, some vegetables, dairy products and seafood will lose their flavor and texture if simmered for too long, so if the recipe calls for including them near the end of the process, be sure to follow the directions carefully.

Crock Pot Benefits

The Crock Pot tge current must-have kitchen appliance. It's not surprising either, the benefits of using a crockpot are plenty! They have several noteworthy features.

- ✓ The broadened cooking times permit better appropriation of flavors across several recipes.
- ✓ The lower temperatures reduce the chance that your foods will burn compared to conventional stove or oven cooking.
- ✓ More affordable or tough meats, for example, chunk steaks or roast and less lean stewing beef, are tenderized through the long cooking process.
- ✓ The crockpot liberates your broiler and stove top for different utilizations, and it is an awesome decision for extensive social affairs or occasion dinners. There's no compelling reason to scour a few pots and skillet. As a rule, you'll just need to wash the crockpot and possibly a couple of prep utensils - and so saving lots of your valuable time!
- ✓ Crockpots utilize less power than a standard electric broiler. The crockpot won't warm the kitchen up the way a huge stove will, however.

✓ A crockpot transports well. Take it from your kitchen to the workplace or gathering. Simply connect it to power and serve.

✓ A crockpot meal is an efficient decision for a bustling day, regardless of whether you work in or out of your home.

Is the Crock Pot safe?

Crockpots are designed to cook for several hours at a time and heat food properly, but you should still practice some safety precautions.

✓ Never fill the stoneware container more than two-thirds full and keep the lid on throughout the cooking process to maintain ideal cooking conditions inside the container.

✓ Periodically, you should test the cooker to make sure the unit heats correctly and is able to cook food to a proper serving temperature. Food should cook to at least 140 degrees Fahrenheit (60 degrees Celsius) within four hours to avoid harboring bacteria.

✓ To test your slow cooker, fill it one-half to two-thirds with water, cover it with the lid, and cook on the low setting for eight hours. Then, use a food thermometer to monitor the water temperature before it cools. If the temperature is 185 degrees Fahrenheit (85 degrees Celsius) or higher, the slow cooker is safe to use. A lower temperature may indicate that the heating element isn't functioning well enough to cook food thoroughly.

Slow cookers run off a low wattage, so it's safe to leave the house while it's on. Although the base does heat up, the product is designed to not get so hot that it'll set a countertop on fire. Never immerse the base of a slow cooker in water. If your slow cooker doesn't have a removable insert, use a soapy sponge to clean the inside and wipe away any spills.

Crock Pot

RECIPES

Ham Broccoli Cheese Casserole

Calories: 209 Carbs: 5 g Fat: 18g Protein: 11g
Servings: 8
Cooking: 1-3 hours

Ingredients:
- ½ diced yellow onion
- 16 ounces broccoli florets
- 1 C./250 ml diced ham
- Pepper and salt
- 1/3 C./75 ml shredded parmesan cheese
- 1 ½ C./350 ml shredded cheddar cheese
- 1 C./250 ml/250 ml heavy cream
- 10 beaten eggs
- 1 tbsp./15 ml butter

Preparation:
1. Liberally grease the bottom of your crockpot with butter.
2. Pour ½ cup of cheddar cheese, heavy cream, parmesan cheese, eggs and a few dashes of pepper and salt into the pot.
3. Whisk well and then stir in the onion, broccoli and ham.
4. Sprinkle with the remaining cheddar cheese.
5. Set to cook on high for 1-3 hours.

Poblano Cheese Frittata

Calories: 257 Carbs: 6g Fat: 19g Protein: 14g
Servings: 4
Cooking: 1-2 hours

Ingredients:
- ¼ C./ 60 ml chopped cilantro
- 1 C./250 ml Mexican blended shredded cheese
- ½ tsp./2.5 ml cumin
- ½ -1 tsp./15 ml salt
- 10-ounce can green chilies
- 1 C./250 ml half and halt
- 4 eggs

Preparation:
1. Slice the chilies.
2. Beat in the eggs and mix them together with ½ cup of shredded cheese, cumin, salt – half and half.
3. Pour the mixture into a pan. With foil, cover the pan.
4. Place a trivet into the bottom of the crockpot and gently set the pan on top. Pour 1 cup of water into the pot.
5. Set to cook on high for 1-2 hours.
6. When done, sprinkle the remaining shredded cheese over the top.
7. Stick it into a broiler for 5 minutes to melt.
8. Serve and enjoy!

Broccoli Ham and Pepper Frittata

Calories: 422 Carbs: 9g Fat: 30g Protein: 28g
Servings: 4
Cooking: 1 – 1 ½ hours

Ingredients:

- ✓ 2 tsp./30 ml pepper
- ✓ 1 tsp./15 ml salt
- ✓ 1 C./250 ml shredded cheddar cheese
- ✓ 1 C./250 ml half and half
- ✓ 2 C. 500 ml frozen broccoli
- ✓ 4 eggs
- ✓ 1 C./250 ml sliced sweet peppers
- ✓ 8 ounces cubed ham

Preparation:

1. Liberally grease a pan.
2. Arrange the peppers into the bottom of the pan.
3. Layer the cubed ham over the top, then the broccoli.
4. Whisk the pepper, salt, half and half, and eggs together. Stir in the cheese and pour over the broccoli mixture.
5. Cover the pan with foil.
6. Place a trivet into the crockpot, pour in 1 cup water around it and place the pan upon the trivet.
7. Set to cook on high for 1-1 ½ hours.
8. If you desire, sprinkle more cheese over top and place in a broiler 5 minutes to melt.
9. Serve and Enjoy!

Sous Vide Bacon Egg Bites

Calories: 124 Carbs: 3g Fat: 8g Protein: 9g
Servings: 9
Cooking: 1 hour

Ingredients:

- ✓ 1 C./250 ml shredded cheese
- ✓ 1 C./250 ml chopped red onion
- ✓ ½ chopped green pepper
- ✓ ½ chopped red pepper
- ✓ ¼ C./60 ml heavy whipping cream
- ✓ ½ C./ 125 ml cottage cheese
- ✓ 4 slices of cooked and crumbled bacon
- ✓ ¼ C./60 ml egg whites
- ✓ 4 eggs

Preparation:

1. In a blender, add the pepper, salt, cheese, whipping cream, cottage cheese, egg whites, and eggs. Blend for 30-45 seconds till well incorporated.
2. Add a trivet into the crockpot and pour in 1 cup of water.
3. Ladle the egg mixture into baby food jars. Then place them on a trivet.
4. Top with bacon, onions, and peppers.
5. Set to cook on high for 1 hour.
6. To take out the bits from the jars, push on the bottom of each one.
7. Serve and enjoy!

Overnight Breakfast Casserole

Calories: 256 Carbs: 5g Fat: 19g Protein: 15g
Servings: 8-12
Cooking: 4 hours

Ingredients:

- ✓ 1/8 tsp./.25ml sweetener of choice
- ✓ ¼ tsp./1.25ml pepper
- ✓ ½ tsp./2.5ml salt
- ✓ ½ C./125ml unsweetened almond milk
- ✓ 12 eggs
- ✓ 1 diced red pepper
- ✓ 1 diced green pepper
- ✓ 1 diced onion
- ✓ 1 C./250 ml shredded mozzarella cheese
- ✓ 2 C./500ml shredded cheddar cheese
- ✓ 1 pound cooked and chopped bacon
- ✓ ½ pound ground sausage

Preparation:

1. Liberally grease the inside of your crockpot.
2. Add half of the red pepper, green pepper, onion, cheese, bacon, and half of the sausage. Repeat layers till you use all ingredients.
3. Whisk sweetener, pepper, salt, milk, and eggs together. Pour over cheese layers.
4. Set to cook on high for 4 hours.

Mexican Breakfast Casserole

Calories: 320 Carbs: 5g Fat: 24g Protein: 17g
Servings: 10
Cooking: 5 hours

Ingredients:

- ✓ 1 C./250 ml pepper jack cheese
- ✓ 1 C./250 ml unsweetened almond milk
- ✓ 10 eggs
- ✓ 1 C./250 ml salsa
- ✓ ¼ tsp./1.25ml pepper
- ✓ ¼ tsp./1.25ml salt
- ✓ 1 tsp./5ml chili powder
- ✓ 1 tsp./5ml cumin
- ✓ ½ tsp./2.5ml coriander
- ✓ ½ tsp./2.5ml garlic powder
- ✓ 12 ounces pork sausage roll

Preparation:

1. Cook the pork sausage in a skillet till no pink color remains. Add the salsa and seasonings, combining well.
2. Whisk the milk and eggs together.
3. Mix the pork and eggs together.
4. Stir in the cheese and incorporate well.
5. Grease the bottom of your crockpot. Pour the mixture into the pot.
6. Set to cook on low for 5 hours or set to cook on low for 2 ½ hours.
7. Top with your favorite toppings and enjoy!

Cauliflower Casserole

Calories: 189 Carbs: 2g Fat: 17g Protein: 11g
Servings: 5-7
Cooking: 5-7 hours

Ingredients:

- ✓ 2 C./500ml shredded cheddar cheese
- ✓ 1 pound breakfast sausage, cooked
- ✓ 1 head cauliflower, shredded
- ✓ ½ tsp./2.5ml pepper
- ✓ 1 tsp./15ml salt
- ✓ ½ tsp./2.5ml dry mustard
- ✓ ½ C./125ml unsweetened almond milk
- ✓ 12 eggs
- ✓ 1 diced onion

Preparation:

1. Grease your crockpot.
2. Beat the pepper, salt, dry mustard, milk and eggs together.
3. Pour 1/3 of the shredded cauliflower mixture into the crockpot and top with 1/3 of diced onion. Season with pepper and salt. Then top with 1/3 of sausage and 1/3 of cheese. Repeat the layers till you use all your ingredients.
4. Pour the mixture over the layers.
5. Set to cook on low for 5-7 hours.
6. Serve and Enjoy!

Ham and Egg Casserole

Calories: 276 Carbs: 3g Fat: 28g Protein: 15g
Servings: 4
Cooking: 1 hour

Ingredients:

- ✓ ½ C./125ml heavy cream
- ✓ 6 eggs
- ✓ 1 C./250 ml shredded cheese
- ✓ 2 chopped green onions
- ✓ 1 trimmed ham steak, chopped into cubes
- ✓ 1 tbsp./15ml butter

Preparation:

1. Place the butter into the crockpot, turn it on low to melt.
2. Add the green onions and cubed ham to the pot.
3. Beat the cream and eggs together and pour over the ham and onions.
4. Add the cheese and season with pepper. Stir well to incorporate.
5. Set to cook on high for 1 hour.

Breakfast Pie

Calories: 167 Carbs: 2g Fat: 17g Protein: 9g
Servings: 4-10
Cooking: 6-8 hours

Ingredients:

- ✓ 2 tsp./10ml dried basil
- ✓ 1 tbsp./30ml garlic powder
- ✓ 1 diced yellow onion
- ✓ 1 pound pork breakfast sausage
- ✓ 1 shredded sweet potato
- ✓ 8 whisked eggs
- ✓ Veggies of choice, such as squash, peppers, etc.

Preparation:

1. Grease your crockpot.
2. Shred the potato.
3. Place all the ingredients into your crockpot and stir well to combine.
4. Set to cook on low for 6-8 hours.
5. Slice the mixture into pie wedges and devour!

Egg and Sausage Casserole

Calories: 381 Carbs: 2g Fat: 32g Protein: 20g
Servings: 9
Cooking: 5-6 hours

Ingredients:

- ✓ 6 eggs
- ✓ 2 C./500ml shredded cheese
- ✓ 1 C./250 ml unsweetened almond milk
- ✓ 1-pound sausage

Preparation:

1. Grease your crockpot.
2. In a skillet, brown the sausage.
3. Beat the milk and eggs together.
4. Season with pepper and salt.
5. Pour the mixture into a greased crockpot.
6. Set to cook on low for 5-6 hours.
7. Serve and enjoy!

Turkey Stuffed Peppers

Calories: 124 Carbs: 3g Fat: 8g Protein: 9g
Servings: 4
Cooking: 6-8 hours

Ingredients:

- ✓ ½ C./125ml water
- ✓ 24-ounce jar low-carb pasta sauce
- ✓ 4 green bell peppers
- ✓ 1 minced garlic clove
- ✓ 1 peeled and diced onion
- ✓ 1 pound ground turkey
- ✓ 1 tbsp./15ml olive oil

Preparation:

1. Mix 2 tablespoons of pasta sauce with garlic, onion and turkey. Divide the mixture into 4 equal portions.
2. Slice the tops off the peppers and remove the innards.
3. Place the turkey mixture portions into the peppers.
4. Coat the crockpot with olive oil and place the peppers into the pot. Top with the remaining pasta sauce.
5. Pour water carefully around the peppers
6. Set to cook on low for 6-8 hours.
7. Serve and enjoy!

Salsa and Cheese Crockpot Chicken

Calories: 306 Carbs: 5g Fat: 21g Protein: 14g
Servings: 6
Cooking: 2 ½ hours

Ingredients:

- ✓ 1 ½ C./350ml shredded cheese
- ✓ 1 ½ C./350ml salsa (preferably fresh)
- ✓ 1 ½ pounds boneless, skinless chicken, your choice of cut

Preparation:

1. With olive oil, grease your crockpot.
2. Place a cut of chicken into the crockpot and top with salsa.
3. Set to cook on high for 2 hours.
4. Ensure your oven is preheated to 425 degrees.
5. Put the chicken on a greased sheet. Use the salsa from the pot to cover the chicken. Top with cheese.
6. Bake for 15 minutes.
7. Serve garnished with sour cream and cilantro if you desire.

Turkey Taco Lettuce Wraps

Calories: 210 Carbs: 1g Fat: 11g Protein: 18g
Servings: 4
Cooking: 6-8 hours

Ingredients:

- ✓ ½ C./125ml chicken broth
- ✓ ½ tsp./2.5ml red pepper
- ✓ 8 ounces tomato sauce
- ✓ ½ tsp./2.5ml cumin
- ✓ 2 tbsp./30ml chili powder
- ✓ 2 cloves garlic
- ✓ ½ C./125ml chopped onion
- ✓ 1 pound ground turkey

Preparation:

1. Mix all the recipe ingredients together till well incorporated.
2. Pour the mix into your crockpot.
3. Set to cook on low for 6-8 hours.
4. Serve in lettuce wraps!

Garlic Chicken Drumsticks

Calories: 378 Carbs: 2g Fat: 12g Protein: 22g
Servings: 4
Cooking: 6-8 hours

Ingredients:

- ✓ 1 C./250 ml chicken broth
- ✓ 6 whole garlic cloves
- ✓ 1 tsp./5ml paprika
- ✓ ¼ C./60ml olive oil
- ✓ 8 chicken legs
- ✓ 1 C./250 ml thinly sliced onion

Preparation:

1. Mix together all the ingredients till well combined.
2. Pour the mix into your crockpot.
3. Set to cook on low for 6-8 hours.
4. Enjoy!

Chicken Tacos

Calories: 246 Carbs: 4g Fat: 18g Protein: 24g
Servings: 6-8
Cooking: 8-10 hours

Ingredients:

- ✓ 1 diced onion
- ✓ 15-ounce can diced tomatoes
- ✓ 1 packet of taco seasoning
- ✓ 3-4 boneless, skinless chicken breasts

Preparation:

1. Put the chicken in the bottom of your crockpot. Sprinkle with taco seasoning.
2. Pour the can of tomatoes over the chicken.
3. Then sprinkle the onion over everything and close the lid.
4. Set to cook on low for 8-10 hours.
5. With forks, shred chicken and stir well with the ingredients it cooked with.
6. Cook for another 10 minutes to heat everything through well.
7. Eat on tortillas!

Pork Carnitas

Calories: 321 Carbs: 6g Fat: 19g Protein: 27g
Servings: 6
Cooking: 7-8 hours

Ingredients:

- ✓ ½ C./125ml water
- ✓ ½ C./125ml taco sauce
- ✓ 2 bay leaves
- ✓ 1 tbsp./15ml cumin
- ✓ 2 tbsp./30ml chili powder
- ✓ 2 crushed and minced garlic cloves
- ✓ 1 sliced red pepper
- ✓ 1 sliced orange pepper
- ✓ 1 sliced yellow pepper
- ✓ 1 diced onion
- ✓ 3 pounds of boneless pork chops

Preparation:

1. Pour water into your crockpot. Add the pork chops.
2. Add the remaining ingredients into the pot and stir well to combine.
3. Set to cook on low for 7-8 hours or set to cook on high for 5-6 hours.
4. With forks, shred meat.
5. Serve and Enjoy!

Italian Beef

Calories: 390 Carbs: 6g Fat: 32g Protein: 24g
Servings: 6
Cooking: 10 hours

Ingredients:

- ✓ 1 ½ C./350ml beef broth
- ✓ 1 sliced onion
- ✓ 1 tbsp./15ml Italian seasoning
- ✓ 1 boneless beef chuck roast
- ✓ 12-ounce jar whole pepperoncini

Preparation:

1. Put the beef roast into a freezer bag.
2. Pour in the whole jar of pepperoncinis with the liquid.
3. Add onion and Italian seasoning. Let it marinate for 1-2 hours.
4. Pour the contents of your freezer bag into the crockpot.
5. Set to cook on low for 10 hours.
6. Shred with forks and serve with onions and peppers.

Roasted Red Pepper Chicken

Calories: 213 Carbs: 1g Fat: 17g Protein: 19g
Servings: 4
Cooking: 6-8 hours

Ingredients:

- ✓ 1 C./250 ml chicken broth
- ✓ ½ tsp./2.5ml cumin
- ✓ ½ - 1 tsp./5ml red pepper flakes
- ✓ ½ -1 tsp./5ml chili powder
- ✓ 24-ounce jar roasted red peppers
- ✓ ¼ C./60ml olive oil
- ✓ 4 crushed and minced garlic cloves
- ✓ 1 seeded and chopped green pepper
- ✓ ½ C./125ml chopped onion
- ✓ 4-6 boneless, skinless chicken thighs

Preparation:

1. Mix together all the ingredients in your crockpot.
2. Set to cook on low for 6-8 hours.
3. Serve and Enjoy!

Shrimp Fajitas

Calories: 328 Carbs: 6g Fat: 21g Protein: 29g
Servings: 4
Cooking: 2 hours

Ingredients:

- ✓ 1 tsp./5ml salt
- ✓ ½ tsp./2.5ml paprika
- ✓ 1 tsp./5ml chili powder
- ✓ 1 packet of taco seasoning
- ✓ ½ C./125ml chicken broth
- ✓ 1 pound deveined and peeled raw shrimp
- ✓ 1 sliced onion
- ✓ 1 quartered tomato
- ✓ 2 sliced red peppers
- ✓ 2 sliced green peppers

Preparation:

1. Pour all the ingredients into your crockpot, minus the shrimp.
2. Set to cook on low for 2 hours.
3. Enjoy!

Steak Bites

Calories: 275 Carbs: 1g Fat: 16g Protein: 23g
Servings: 4
Cooking: 6-8 hours

Ingredients:

- ✓ 4 tbsp./60ml butter
- ✓ ½ tsp./2.5ml pepper
- ✓ ½ tsp./2.5ml salt
- ✓ 1 tsp./5ml garlic powder
- ✓ 1 tbsp./15ml minced onion
- ✓ ½ C./125ml beef broth
- ✓ 3-4 pound round steak

Preparation:

1. Cut the steak into 1-inch cubes. Place the cubes inside your crockpot.
2. Pour the broth over the cubes.
3. Sprinkle the meat with pepper, salt, garlic powder and minced onion.
4. Slice the butter and place slices over the top.
5. Set to cook on low for 6-8 hours or set to cook on high for 3-4 hours.
6. Serve & Enjoy!

Unstuffed Pepper Soup

Calories: 202 Carbs: 1g Fat: 10g Protein: 19g
Servings: 4
Cooking: 6-8 hours

Ingredients:

- ✓ 2 C./500ml water
- ✓ 1 pound ground beef
- ✓ 2 tsp./10ml Italian seasoning
- ✓ 2 tbsp./30ml coconut aminos
- ✓ 2 10-ounce cans Rotel
- ✓ 8-ounce can no-sugar-added tomato sauce
- ✓ 2 crushed garlic cloves
- ✓ 1 seeded and diced yellow pepper
- ✓ 1 seeded and diced orange pepper
- ✓ 1 seeded and diced green pepper
- ✓ 1 seeded and diced red pepper
- ✓ 1 C./250 ml diced onion

Preparation:

1. Mix together all the ingredients.
2. Pour the mixture into your crockpot.
3. Set to cook on low for 6-8 hours.
4. Serve & Enjoy!

Jalapeno Popper Chicken Soup

Calories: 289 Carbs: 6g Fat: 20g Protein: 14g
Servings: 6
Cooking: 3-4 hours

Ingredients:

- ✓ 1 chopped jalapeno pepper
- ✓ 8 ounces cream cheese
- ✓ ½ pound bacon
- ✓ 1 C./250 ml water
- ✓ 1 can cream of chicken soup
- ✓ ¼ chopped onion
- ✓ 2 seeded/chopped jalapeno peppers
- ✓ 2 tbsp./30ml taco seasoning
- ✓ 1 tsp./5ml pepper
- ✓ 1 tsp./5ml salt
- ✓ 3 boneless chicken breasts

Preparation:

1. Put the chicken into the bottom of your crockpot.
2. Sprinkle with taco seasoning, pepper and salt. Then add water, cream of chicken soup, onions and jalapenos. Stir well to incorporate.
3. Set to cook on low for 6-8 hours or set to cook on high for 3-4 hours.
4. Shred the chicken and add it back to the pot.
5. Cube the cream cheese and stir it into the soup till it melts.
6. Fry the bacon, chop it up and add it to the soup.
7. Serve with additional bacon, jalapeno peppers, cheddar cheese, sour cream, and so on.

Chicken Bacon Chowder

Calories: 355 Carbs: 6g Fat: 28g Protein: 21g
Servings: 8
Cooking: 6-8 hours

Ingredients:

- ✓ 1 tsp./5ml thyme
- ✓ 1 tsp./5ml garlic powder
- ✓ 1 tsp./5ml pepper
- ✓ 1 tsp./5ml sea salt
- ✓ 1 pound cooked and crumbled bacon
- ✓ 1 C./250 ml heavy cream
- ✓ 8 ounces cream cheese
- ✓ 1 pound chicken breasts
- ✓ 2 C./500ml chicken stock
- ✓ 4 tbsp./60ml butter
- ✓ 1 thinly sliced sweet onion
- ✓ 6 ounces sliced cremini mushrooms
- ✓ 2 diced celery ribs
- ✓ 1 trimmed and sliced leek
- ✓ 1 chopped shallot
- ✓ 4 minced garlic cloves

Preparation:

1. Turn your crockpot to low.
2. Add the pepper, salt, 1 cup of stock, 2 tablespoons of butter, onions, mushrooms, leek, celery, shallot and garlic.
3. Cover and cook for 1 hour to soften the veggies.
4. While the veggies cook, pan sear the chicken breasts with the remaining butter.
5. Set the chicken to the side and deglaze the pan with the remaining chicken stock.
6. Scrape up the cooking bits and add the deglazed stock mixture to the crockpot.
7. Add the thyme, garlic powder, cream cheese,and heavy cream to pot. Stir well to combine.
8. Cut the chicken into cubes once cooled and add them to the pot. Stir in the bacon.
9. Set to cook on low for 6-8 hours.

Zuppa Toscana Soup

Calories: 246 Carbs: 7g Fat: 19g Protein: 14g
Servings: 10
Cooking: 8 hours

Ingredients:

- ✓ ½ C./125ml heavy cream
- ✓ ½ tsp./2.5ml pepper
- ✓ 1 tsp./5ml salt
- ✓ ¼ tsp./1.25ml crushed red pepper flakes
- ✓ 3 C./750ml chopped kale
- ✓ 1 diced cauliflower head
- ✓ 36-ounces chicken stock
- ✓ 3 minced garlic cloves
- ✓ ½ C./125ml finely diced onion
- ✓ 1 tbsp./15ml olive oil
- ✓ 1 pound ground Italian sausage

Preparation:

1. Brown the sausage in a pan. Remove it from the pan into your crockpot.
2. Pour the oil into a skillet. Sauté the onions for 3-4 minutes till softened.
3. Add the sautéed onions, pepper, salt, red pepper flakes, kale, cauliflower florets and chicken stock to the pot.
4. Set to cook on high for 4 hours or set to cook on low for 8 hours.
5. Add the heavy cream at the end, stirring well to incorporate.

Taco Soup

Calories: 219 Carbs: 2g Fat: 14g Protein: 9g
Servings: 8
Cooking: 6-8 hours

Ingredients:

- ✓ 2 tsp./10ml salt
- ✓ 1 tsp./5ml onion powder
- ✓ 1 tbsp./15ml chili powder
- ✓ 1 tbsp./15ml cumin
- ✓ 3 tbsp./45ml chopped garlic
- ✓ 1 diced onion
- ✓ 1 can Rotel
- ✓ 1 package cream cheese
- ✓ 4 C./1l bone broth
- ✓ 2 C./500ml water
- ✓ 2 pounds ground beef

Preparation:

1. Pour all the ingredients into your crockpot.
2. Set to cook on low for 6-8 hours.
3. Stir 1-2 times during cooking.
4. Serve topped any keto-friendly topping.

Bacon Cheeseburger Soup

Calories: 359 Carbs: 4g Fat: 16g Protein: 21g
Servings: 8
Cooking: 1 hour

Ingredients:

- ✓ ½ C./125ml heavy cream
- ✓ 3 ounces cream cheese
- ✓ 1 C./250 ml shredded cheddar cheese
- ✓ 3 diced dill pickles
- ✓ 2 ½ tbsp./22.5ml tomato paste
- ✓ 1 tsp./5ml chili powder
- ✓ 1 tsp./5ml cumin
- ✓ ½ tsp./2.5ml ground red pepper
- ✓ ½ tsp./2.5ml pepper
- ✓ 2 tbsp./30ml yellow mustard
- ✓ ½ tsp./2.5ml onion powder
- ✓ ½ tsp./2.5ml garlic powder
- ✓ 3 C./750ml beef broth
- ✓ 2 tbsp./30ml butter
- ✓ 12 ounces ground beef
- ✓ 5 slices of bacon

Preparation:

1. Cook the bacon.
2. Take it out of the pan and brown the beef in the same pan in the bacon grease.
3. Add the spices and butter to another pan. Cook for 45 seconds. Add the cream cheese, mustard, cheese, tomato paste and broth to the butter and spice mixture.
4. Cook for 5 minutes to melt the cream cheese.
5. Add the pickles and heavy cream to the sauce.
6. Pour the sauce over the meat and simmer for 5-10 minutes.
7. Pour everything into your crockpot. Set to cook on high for 1 hour.
8. Serve & Enjoy!

Pizza Soup

Calories: 405 Carbs: 4g Fat: 31g Protein: 18g
Servings: 8
Cooking: 4-5 hours

Ingredients:

- ✓ 1 C./250 ml mini pepperonis
- ✓ 1 tbsp./15ml Italian seasoning
- ✓ 2.25-ounce can black olives, drained
- ✓ 4 ounces mushrooms
- ✓ 16 ounces cream cheese
- ✓ 1 C./250 ml water
- ✓ 14.5-ounce can beef broth
- ✓ 2 C./500ml marinara sauce
- ✓ 1-2 pounds browned ground sausage

Preparation:

1. In your crockpot, combine all the ingredients till well incorporated.
2. Set to cook on low for 4-5 hours or set to cook on high for 2-3 hours.
3. Serve topped with mozzarella cheese if you so choose.

Creamy Garlic Chicken Soup

Calories: 307 Carbs: 2g Fat: 25g Protein: 18g
Servings: 4
Cooking: 1 ½ hours

Ingredients:

- ✓ ¼ C./60ml heavy cream
- ✓ 14.5 ounces chicken broth
- ✓ 2 tbsp./30ml garlic gusto seasoning
- ✓ 4 ounces cream cheese
- ✓ 2 C./500ml shredded chicken
- ✓ 2 tbsp./30ml butter

Preparation:

1. Melt the butter in your crockpot. Add the chicken.
2. As the chicken starts to warm, add in the cream cheese and gusto seasoning. Mix well till combined.
3. Set to cook on high for 1 ½ hours.
4. Enjoy!

Green Chili Enchilada Soup

Calories: 278 Carbs: 5g Fat: 19g Protein: 11g
Servings: 8
Cooking: 7 hours

Ingredients:

- ✓ 8 ounces softened cream cheese
- ✓ 1 tsp./15ml garlic powder
- ✓ 1 tsp./15ml onion powder
- ✓ 2 tbsp./30ml cumin
- ✓ ¾ C. /175mlwater
- ✓ 4-ounce can diced green chilies
- ✓ 15-ounce jar salsa
- ✓ 24 ounces chicken breasts
- ✓ 32 ounces chicken broth

Preparation:

1. Put the chicken into the bottom of the crockpot. Add the cumin, onion powder, garlic powder, chili powder, water, salsa, green chilies and broth over the chicken. Stir well to incorporate.
2. Set to cook on low for 7 hours.
3. Mix in the cream cheese, stirring till dissolved. Cook for an additional half an hour to heat the soup.

Lasagna Soup

Calories: 391 Carbs: 2g Fat: 25g Protein: 18g
Servings: 8
Cooking: 2 hours

Ingredients:

- ✓ 5-6 basil leaves
- ✓ ½ C./125ml shredded parmesan cheese
- ✓ 1 C./250 ml shredded mozzarella cheese
- ✓ ½ C./125ml heavy whipping cream
- ✓ 2 C./500ml beef broth
- ✓ 1 tsp./5ml garlic salt
- ✓ 1 C./250 ml cottage cheese
- ✓ 1 tsp./5ml paprika
- ✓ 2 tsp./10ml red pepper flakes
- ✓ 1 tbsp./15ml Italian blend herbs
- ✓ 2 14.5-ounce cans fire roasted tomatoes
- ✓ 1 diced sweet onion
- ✓ 2 diced garlic cloves
- ✓ 1 tbsp./15ml Italian sausage seasoning
- ✓ 2-pound ground pork

Preparation:

1. Pour the seasonings, tomatoes, garlic, onion, and meat into your crockpot. Set to cook on high for 2 hours.
2. Break up the meat.
3. Add the cottage cheese to a blender, blending till liquefied. Add to the soup.
4. Set the pot to low till you are ready to devour!

Old Fashioned Beef Stew

Calories: 253 Carbs:32g Fat: 19g Protein: 9g
Servings: 8
Cooking: 6 hours

Ingredients:

- ✓ 1 package mixed veggies
- ✓ 1 bay leaf
- ✓ 1 tsp./5ml salt
- ✓ ½ tsp./2.5ml garlic powder
- ✓ 3 tbsp./45ml Worcestershire sauce
- ✓ 28-ounce can tomato sauce
- ✓ 4 C./1l beef broth
- ✓ 1 C./250 ml honeyville almond flour
- ✓ 1 package of stew meat
- ✓ 2 tbsp./30ml olive oil

Preparation:

1. Warm the olive oil in a skillet.
2. Add the flour and stew the meat. Coat the meat.
3. Cook for 5-10 minutes till evenly browned.
4. Add the stew meat to the crockpot, along with the cooking bits from the skillet.
5. Add the remaining ingredients to the pot.
6. Set to cook on high for 6 hours.
7. Discard the bay leaf and serve!

Brunswick Stew

Calories: 437 Carbs: 11g Fat: 20g Protein: 21g
Servings: 10
Cooking: 5-6 hours

Ingredients:

- ✓ 5 C./1.25l beef broth
- ✓ 2 peeled and cubed sweet potatoes (keto friendly)
- ✓ 18-ounces BBQ sauce
- ✓ 28-ounce can crushed tomatoes
- ✓ 1 diced onion
- ✓ 2 pounds ground beef

Preparation:

1. Brown and crumble up the beef in a skillet along with the onion.
2. Peel and cube the sweet potatoes as the meat cooks.
3. Drain the grease from the beef.
4. Add all the ingredients to the crockpot. Stir to incorporate thoroughly.
5. Set to cook on high for 3 hours or set to cook on low for 5-6 hours.

Beef Cabbage Stew

Calories: 489 Carbs: 5g Fat: 28g Protein: 41g
Servings: 8-10
Cooking: 5 hours

Ingredients:

- ✓ 8-ounce can tomato sauce
- ✓ 8-ounce can whole plum tomatoes
- ✓ 5 sliced celery stalks
- ✓ 8 ounces shredded cabbage
- ✓ 2 bay leaves
- ✓ ¼ tsp./1.25ml Pepper
- ✓ 1 tsp./5ml Greek seasoning
- ✓ 2 chopped onion
- ✓ 1 1/3 C./75 ml hot chicken broth
- ✓ 1 beef bouillon cube
- ✓ 2 pounds beef stew meat

Preparation:

1. In a pan, brown the stew meat for 5 minutes. Drain the grease.
2. Stir a boullion cube into the broth until it is dissolved.
3. Add the bay leaves, pepper, Greek seasoning and onions to the broth mixture.
4. Add the stew meat and broth mixture to the crockpot. Stir well to combine.
5. Set to cook on low for 7 hours or set to cook on high for 4 ½ - 5 hours.
6. Stir in the cabbage.
7. Trash the bay leaves before serving the stew

Beef and Sweet Potato Stew

Calories: 396 Carbs: 6g Fat: 29g Protein: 21g
Servings: 8
Cooking: 4-6 hours

Ingredients:

- ✓ 4 tbsp./60ml chopped parsley
- ✓ 2 bay leaves
- ✓ 1 tsp./5ml paprika
- ✓ ½ tsp./2.5ml pepper
- ✓ ½ - 1 tsp./5ml salt
- ✓ 1 crushed beef bouillon cube
- ✓ 14-ounce can diced tomatoes
- ✓ 1 ½ C./350ml beef broth
- ✓ 10 ounce halved sweet potatoes (keto friendly)
- ✓ 2 sliced carrots
- ✓ 4 crushed garlic cloves
- ✓ 1/3 C./75 ml honeyville almond flour
- ✓ 3 pounds beef stew meat
- ✓ 1 sweet potato

Preparation:

1. Pour the flour and stew meat into your crockpot. Stir well to the coat meat.
2. Add the remaining ingredients into the pot, minus parsley and bay leaves.
3. Stir well to incorporate thoroughly. Add bay leaves to the top.
4. Set to cook on low for 8-10 hours or set to cook on high for 4-6 hours.
5. Season with pepper and salt, discard the bay leaves.
6. Serve garnished with parsley.

Double Beef Stew

Calories: 222 Carbs: 11g Fat: 7g Protein: 27g
Servings: 6
Cooking: 2 hours

Ingredients:

- ✓ 1 tbsp./15ml Worcestershire sauce
- ✓ 2 tsp./10ml hot sauce
- ✓ 1 C./250 ml beef broth
- ✓ 1 tbsp./15 ml chili mix
- ✓ 2 14.5-ounce cans diced tomatoes
- ✓ 5 pounds beef stew meat

Preparation:

1. Set your crockpot to high.
2. Pour all the ingredients into the pot and stir well to combine.
3. Set to cook for 6 hours on high.
4. Break up the meat and pull it apart with a fork.
5. Season if needed.
6. Set to cook for 2 hours on low.
7. Devour!

Chicken Stew

Calories: 228 Carbs: 6g Fat: 11g Protein: 23g
Servings: 4
Cooking: 4 hours

Ingredients:

- ✓ ½ C./125ml heavy cream
- ✓ ½ tsp./2.5ml dried oregano
- ✓ ¼ tsp./1.25ml dried thyme
- ✓ 1 sprig rosemary
- ✓ 28 ounces skinless, deboned chicken thighs sliced into 1-inch pieces
- ✓ 1 C./250 ml diced celery
- ✓ ½ C./125ml peeled and diced carrots
- ✓ 2 C./500ml chicken stock
- ✓ 1 C./250 ml spinach

Preparation:

1. Add the oregano, thyme, garlic, rosemary, chicken thighs, onion, celery, carrots and chicken stock to your crockpot.
2. Set to cook on high for 2 hours or set to cook on low for 4 hours.
3. Mix in the spinach and heavy cream.
4. Whisk for 10 minutes till it becomes a bit thicker.
5. Tip! You can use a bit of xanthan gum to help stew thicken more.

Autumn Beef and Veggie Stew

Calories: 553 Carbs: 9g Fat: 39g Protein: 31g
Servings: 8-10
Cooking: 6 hours

Ingredients:

- ✓ 4-5 zucchinis
- ✓ 1 rutabaga
- ✓ 1 ½ tsp./5.5ml salt
- ✓ 2 cinnamon sticks
- ✓ 2 bay leaves
- ✓ 1 tsp./5ml turmeric powder
- ✓ 1 tsp./5ml coriander seeds
- ✓ 1 tsp./5ml chili powder
- ✓ 1 tsp./5ml ginger
- ✓ 1 tbsp./15ml paprika
- ✓ 2 tbsp./30ml cumin
- ✓ 1 C./250 ml vegetable stock
- ✓ 14-ounce can chopped tomatoes
- ✓ 4 garlic cloves
- ✓ 1 white onion
- ✓ ½ C./125ml ghee
- ✓ 3 ½ pounds boneless braising steaks

Preparation:

1. Turn your crockpot to high.
2. Pat down the steaks and season them with pepper and salt.
3. Place the steaks into a skillet with ¼ cup of ghee. Sear till just browned lightly. Place them into the crockpot.
4. Peel and dice the garlic and onions. Put them into a pan with the remaining ghee, sautéing till fragrant.
5. Add the turmeric, coriander, chili powder, ginger, cumin, broth, paprika, and tomatoes to the pot. Then add bay leaves and cinnamon sticks.
6. Set to cook on high for 3 hours.
7. Push the meat to one side of the pot.
8. Peel and dice the rutabaga and add it to the crockpot.
9. Add the rutabaga to the other side. Cook for another 60 minutes
10. Dice the zucchini. Add the zucchini to the same side as the rutabaga and mix well to combine with the cooking juices.
11. Discard the bay leaves and cinnamon sticks.
12. Cook for another 2 hours. Once the zucchini and rutabaga are tender to the touch of a fork, the stew is done!

Bacon Cabbage Chuck Beef Stew

Calories: 378 Carbs: 4g Fat: 24g Protein: 28g
Servings: 5
Cooking: 7 hours

Ingredients:

- ✓ 1 C./250 ml beef bone broth
- ✓ 1 sprig thyme
- ✓ 1 head of cabbage
- ✓ 1 peeled and smashed garlic clove
- ✓ 2 peeled and sliced red onions
- ✓ 2-3 pounds chuck roast, cut into 2-inch pieces
- ✓ ½ pound uncured bacon, sliced into strips

Preparation:

1. Place the slices of bacon into the bottom of the crockpot.
2. Add the garlic and onion slices to the bacon.
3. Add the roast on top of the onion and garlic.
4. Then add the cabbage slices along with the thyme, broth and a few pinches of pepper and sea salt.
5. Set to cook on low for 7 hours.

Beef and Veggie Stew

Calories: 256 Carbs: 2g Fat: 10g Protein: 14g
Servings: 6-8
Cooking: 4-5 hours

Ingredients:

- ✓ 1 head of cauliflower, sliced in florets
- ✓ 5 C./1.25l beef broth
- ✓ 1/3 C./75 ml honeyville almond flour
- ✓ 1 ½ tsp./5.5ml salt
- ✓ 1 tsp./5ml pepper
- ✓ 2 tsp./10ml minced thyme leaves
- ✓ 2 bay leaves
- ✓ ¼ C./60ml tomato paste
- ✓ 6 minced garlic cloves
- ✓ 6 sliced celery stalks
- ✓ 1 C./250 ml dry white wine
- ✓ 6 ounces white button mushrooms, quartered
- ✓ 1 pound chopped yellow onions
- ✓ 1 pound chopped baby carrots
- ✓ 2 tbsp./30ml extra virgin olive oil
- ✓ 2 pounds beef sirloin tip, cut into ¾-inch cubes

Preparation:

1. Heat up the oil in a pan. Sear the beef cubes until they are browned. Set them to the side.
2. Add the onions, sautéing in the beef grease till fragrant.
3. Add the onions, beef and remaining ingredients to the crockpot. Stir well to incorporate thoroughly. Season with pepper and salt if needed.
4. Set to cook on low for 7-8 hours or set to cook on high for 4-5 hours.
5. Serve garnished with sour cream.

Chunky Beef and Cauliflower Stew

Calories: 413 Carbs: 9g Fat: 39g Protein: 31g
Servings: 4
Cooking: 5 hours

Ingredients:

- ✓ 1 pound of cauliflower, sliced into bite-sized chunks
- ✓ 3 tbsp./45ml honeyville almond flour
- ✓ 2 ½ C./600ml beef stock
- ✓ ½ C. /125ml dry white wine
- ✓ ½ tsp./2.5ml pepper
- ✓ 1 tsp./5ml thyme
- ✓ 1 bay leaf
- ✓ 2 tbsp./30ml tomato paste
- ✓ 3 minced garlic cloves
- ✓ 3 chopped celery stalks
- ✓ 4-ounce can mushrooms
- ✓ 4 chopped carrots
- ✓ 1 chopped onion
- ✓ 1 ¼ pounds beef sirloin tip roast
- ✓ 1 tsp./5ml olive oil

Preparation:

1. Heat up the oil in a pan and sear the beef cubes.
2. Sauté the carrots and onions in the beef grease for 10 minutes until golden.
3. With the white wine, deglaze the pan, removing the cooking bits from the bottom.
4. Add the meat, carrots, onions, cooking bits and all the remaining ingredients to your crockpot. Stir well to incorporate.
5. Set to cook on high for 3 hours or set to cook on low for 5 hours.
6. Enjoy!

5-Ingredient Chili

Calories: 503 Carbs: 6g Fat: 41g Protein: 29g
Servings: 4
Cooking: 2-3 hours

Ingredients:

- ✓ 15 ounces tomato sauce
- ✓ 3-4 cans diced tomatoes
- ✓ 2 diced onions
- ✓ 3-4 pounds meat of choice (ground turkey, bison, sausage, venison, beef, etc.)
- ✓ Cumin and other spices to achieve desired taste, such as cilantro, garlic, salt, chili powder, etc.

Preparation:

1. Pour all the ingredients into your crockpot. Stir well to incorporate.
2. Set to cook on low for 5-6 hours or set to cook on high for 2-3 hours.

Not Your Caveman's Chili

Calories: 390 Carbs: 5g Fat: 16g Protein: 27g
Servings: 4
Cooking: 3 ½ - 4 hours

Ingredients:

- ✓ 1 tsp./5ml salt
- ✓ 1 tsp./5ml pepper
- ✓ 1 tsp./5ml Worcestershire sauce
- ✓ 1 tsp./5ml cayenne pepper
- ✓ 1 tsp./5ml oregano
- ✓ 2 tsp./30ml paprika
- ✓ 2 tsp./30ml minced garlic
- ✓ 2 tsp./30ml fish sauce
- ✓ 1 ½ tsp./5.5ml cumin
- ✓ 2 ½ tbsp./45ml chili powder
- ✓ 2 tbsp./30ml olive oil
- ✓ 2 tbsp./30ml coconut amino sauce
- ✓ 1/3 C./75 ml tomato paste
- ✓ 1 C./250 ml beef broth
- ✓ 1 green pepper
- ✓ 1 onion
- ✓ 2 pounds stew meat

Preparation:

1. Cut half of the stew meat into small cubes. Place the other half into a food processor, blending it into the ground beef.
2. Chop up the onion and pepper into small pieces.
3. Mix together the spices.
4. Sauté the beef in a pan along with the ground beef.
5. Sauté the veggies in the meat grease until fragrant.
6. Add all the other ingredients to your crockpot.
7. Simmer on high for 2 ½ hours. Stir and simmer 20-30 more minutes.

Chocolate Chili

Calories: 492 Carbs: 7g Fat: 25g Protein: 17g
Servings: 4
Cooking: 4 hours

Ingredients:

- ✓ 10 drops liquid stevia
- ✓ 2 tsp./10ml garlic
- ✓ 2 tsp./10ml paprika
- ✓ 1 tsp./5ml cayenne pepper
- ✓ 1 tsp./5ml cumin
- ✓ 1 tbsp./15ml cocoa powder
- ✓ 1 tbsp./15ml chili powder
- ✓ 1 tbsp./15ml coconut amino sauce
- ✓ 2 tbsp./30ml butter
- ✓ 2 tbsp./30ml Worcestershire sauce
- ✓ 2 cans whole tomatoes
- ✓ 1 C./250 ml black coffee
- ✓ 1 C./250 ml beef broth
- ✓ ½ onion
- ✓ 8 ounces kielbasa
- ✓ 6 slices of bacon
- ✓ 2 pounds ground beef

Preparation:

1. Puree both cans of tomatoes in a food processor and add them to your crockpot.
2. Add the spices and all liquid ingredients minus the garlic and butter to the sauce in the crockpot.
3. Add the stevia.
4. Brown the beef in pan. Drain and put to the side.
5. Chop the onion and sauté it in a pan until softened.
6. Add the bacon and kielbasa to the pan with the onions, cooking till the bacon is crispy.
7. Add the sausage and bacon mixture along with the garlic powder to the crockpot.
8. Add the beef to your crockpot.
9. Set to cook on high for 4 hours.

Old-Fashioned Low-Carb Crockpot Chili

Calories: 318 Carbs: 4g Fat: 24g Protein: 17g
Servings: 8
Cooking: 3 hours

Ingredients:

- ✓ 1 tsp./5ml pepper
- ✓ 1 tsp./5ml salt
- ✓ 1 tsp./5ml Italian seasoning
- ✓ 1 tsp./5ml garlic powder
- ✓ 2 tbsp./30ml crushed red pepper flakes
- ✓ 1 tbsp./15ml cumin
- ✓ 3 tbsp./45ml chili powder
- ✓ 6 ounces tomato paste
- ✓ 14.5-ounce can diced tomatoes with green chilies
- ✓ 14.5-ounce can crushed tomatoes
- ✓ 1 C./250 ml beef broth
- ✓ 1 ½ C./350ml diced celery
- ✓ 3 tbsp./45ml minced garlic
- ✓ 1 chopped yellow onion
- ✓ 2 pounds lean ground beef

Preparation:

1. Cook the beef in a pan until browned and drain the grease.
2. Add the garlic to the pan and sauté for 60 seconds.
3. Place the beef into the crockpot. Add the remaining ingredients to the beef. Stir to combine well.
4. Set to cook on low for 6 hours or set to cook on high for 3 hours.
5. Serve & Enjoy!

Creamy White Chicken Chili

Calories: 486 Carbs: 6g Fat: 33g Protein: 39g
Servings: 6
Cooking: 7 hours

Ingredients:

- ✓ ½ C. sour cream
- ✓ 4 ounces cream cheese
- ✓ ½ C. heavy cream
- ✓ 3 tbsp. butter
- ✓ 9 ounces chopped green chilies
- ✓ ½ C. chicken stock
- ✓ 1 tsp. garlic powder
- ✓ 1 tsp. cumin
- ✓ 2 tsp. chili powder
- ✓ 2 pounds chicken

Toppings:

- ✓ 1 C./250 ml shredded pepper jack cheese
- ✓ 1/3 C./75 ml peeled and chopped red onion
- ✓ 1/3 C./75 ml chopped cilantro

Preparation:

1. Place the chicken into the crockpot. Add the green chilies, chicken stock, garlic powder, cumin and chili powder to the chicken.
2. Set to cook on low for 7 hours.
3. 60 minutes before you plan to eat, heat the sour cream, cream cheese, heavy cream and butter together in a pan, stirring till smooth.
4. Shred the chicken.
5. Pour the cream cheese mixture over the chicken, combining well to incorporate.
6. Sprinkle with pepper jack, red onion and cilantro before devouring!

Kickin' Chili

Calories: 137 Carbs: 5g Fat: 15g Protein: 16g
Servings: 6
Cooking: 6-8 hours

Ingredients:

- ✓ 1 bay leaf
- ✓ 1 tsp./5ml pepper
- ✓ 1 tsp./5ml oregano
- ✓ 1 tsp./5ml onion powder
- ✓ 1 tsp./5ml garlic powder
- ✓ ½ tsp./2.5ml cayenne pepper
- ✓ 2 tsp./10ml salt
- ✓ 2 tbsp./30ml cumin
- ✓ 4 tbsp./60ml chili powder
- ✓ 2 tbsp./30ml Worcestershire sauce
- ✓ 14.5-ounce can stewed tomatoes
- ✓ 14.5-ounce can tomatoes with green chilies
- ✓ 6-ounce can tomato paste
- ✓ ¼ C./60ml pickled jalapeno slices
- ✓ 3 diced celery ribs
- ✓ 4 tbsp./60ml minced garlic
- ✓ 1 chopped red onion
- ✓ 2 ½ pounds ground beef

Preparation:

1. Turn the crockpot to low.
2. Brown the beef in a skillet along with the pepper, salt and 2 tablespoons of minced garlic. Drain the excess grease. Pour the beef into the crockpot.
3. Add the remaining ingredients to the crockpot. Stir well to incorporate.
4. Set to cook on low for 6-8 hours.

No Bean Chili

Calories: 201 Carbs: 2g Fat: 19g Protein: 21g
Servings: 6
Cooking: 6-7 hours

Ingredients:

- ✓ 1 C./250 ml water
- ✓ 1 packet of chili seasoning
- ✓ 14.5-ounce can diced tomatoes
- ✓ 14.5-ounce can tomato sauce
- ✓ 2 pounds lean ground beef

Preparation:

1. Cook the ground beef and then add it to your crockpot.
2. Add the remaining ingredients to the pot and stir well to combine.
3. Set to cook on low for 6-7 hours.
4. Serve topped with favorite toppings such as sour cream, cheese, diced onion, etc.
5. Enjoy!

Buffalo Chicken Chili

Calories: 277 Carbs: 11g Fat: 14g Protein: 17g
Servings: 8
Cooking: 8 hours

Ingredients:

- ✓ 8 ounces cream cheese
- ✓ ¼ tsp./1.25ml salt
- ✓ ½ tsp./2.5ml dried cilantro
- ✓ ½ tsp./2.5ml celery salt
- ✓ ½ tsp./2.5ml garlic powder
- ✓ ½ tsp./2.5ml onion powder
- ✓ 1 package of ranch dressing mix
- ✓ ¼ - ½ C./125ml buffalo wing sauce
- ✓ 2 C./500ml chicken broth
- ✓ 14.5-ounce can fire roasted tomatoes
- ✓ 1 pound ground chicken

Preparation:

1. Brown the chicken in a skillet till cooked. Place it into the crockpot.
2. Add the remaining ingredients to the chicken inside the pot. Stir well.
3. Set to cook on high for 4 hours or set to cook on low for 8 hours.
4. Stir well to incorporate the cream cheese and wing sauce throughout the chili mixture.
5. Serve & Enjoy!

Steak Lover's Chili

Calories: 198 Carbs: 6g Fat: 19g Protein: 11g
Servings: 8
Cooking: 6 hours

Ingredients:

- ✓ 1 C./250 ml chicken stock
- ✓ 2 C./500ml canned tomatoes
- ✓ ½ C./125ml sliced leeks
- ✓ 1/8 tsp./.25ml pepper
- ✓ ¼ tsp./1.25ml cayenne pepper
- ✓ ½ tsp./2.5ml salt
- ✓ ½ tsp./2.5ml cumin
- ✓ 1 tbsp./15ml chili powder
- ✓ 2 ½ pounds steak, sliced into 1-inch cubes

Optional Toppings:

- ✓ 1 tsp./5ml cilantro
- ✓ ½ sliced avocado
- ✓ 2 tbsp./30ml sour cream
- ✓ ¼ C./60ml shredded cheddar cheese

Preparation:

1. Pour all the ingredients into your Crock Pot, except for the topping ingredients.
2. Stir well to incorporate. Set to cook on high for 6 hours.
3. Shred the cubes of steak and break up the tomatoes.
4. Serve topped with your desired toppings.

Bacon Chili

Calories: 527 Carbs: 7g Fat: 37g Protein: 51g
Servings: 5
Cooking: 5 hours

Ingredients:

- ✓ 2 C./5ooml chicken stock
- ✓ 1 tsp. /5ml Worcestershire sauce
- ✓ 2 jalapeno peppers
- ✓ 3 garlic cloves
- ✓ 1 tsp./5ml oregano
- ✓ 1 tsp./5ml salt
- ✓ ½ tsp./2.5ml pepper
- ✓ 2 tsp./10ml cumin
- ✓ 1 tbsp./15ml chili powder
- ✓ 5 slices of bacon
- ✓ 1 Roma tomato
- ✓ 1 green bell pepper
- ✓ ¾ white onion
- ✓ 30 ounces lean ground beef

Preparation:

1. Chop up the bacon and add it to a pan. Cook till fat renders out and the bacon is almost cooked.
2. Then add the beef to the pan, cooking till some color forms.
3. Chop up the jalapeno peppers and garlic finely. Roughly chop up the onion, bell pepper and tomato.
4. Add 2 cups of stock to the crockpot along with all the other ingredients. Combine them well.
5. Set to cook on low for 5 hours or set to cook on high for 2 ½ hours.

Cuban Mojo Pork

Calories: 294 Carbs: 7g Fat: 37g Protein: 51g
Servings: 8
Cooking: 6 ½ - 7 hours

Ingredients:

- ✓ ¼ C./60 ml chopped cilantro
- ✓ 2 tsp./10ml cumin
- ✓ 2 tsp./10ml oregano
- ✓ 8 finely cloves of garlic
- ✓ ½ C./125ml olive oil
- ✓ Zest of 1 lime
- ✓ Zest of 1 orange
- ✓ ½ C./125ml lime juice
- ✓ ¾ C./175ml orange juice
- ✓ 1 tsp. /5mlpepper
- ✓ 1 ½ tsp./5.5ml salt
- ✓ 1 bone-in pork shoulder

Preparation:

1. Make a few slits into the pork with a knife.
2. Add all the other ingredients to your crockpot. Mix well to incorporate.
3. Gently place the pork among the other ingredients in the pot. With a spoon, ladle the liquids over the pork.
4. Cover and set to cook on high for 5-6 hours or set to cook on low for 8-10 hours.
5. Remove the pork from your crockpot and place it on a sheet lined with foil.
6. Bake at 400 degrees for 15-20 minutes till browned.
7. Allow to rest for 10-15 minutes before serving!

Crockpot Keto Meatballs

Calories: 171 Carbs: 9g Fat: 17g Protein: 19g
Servings: 14
Cooking: 8 hours

Ingredients:

- ✓ 1 tsp./5ml salt
- ✓ 1 tsp./5ml pepper
- ✓ 2 tbsp./30ml grated parmesan cheese
- ✓ 14 grams crushed pork rinds
- ✓ ¼ C./60ml mayo
- ✓ 1 egg
- ✓ 1 pound ground pork
- ✓ 1 pound ground beef

Sauce:

- ✓ 14-ounce jar chili sauce

Preparation:

1. Turn your crockpot to high. Using olive oil, grease the pot liberally.
2. Combine all the ingredients, minus the sauce ingredients, together well.
3. Roll the mixture into 40-42 meatballs. Place the meatballs into the crockpot.
4. Mix together the sauce ingredients until smooth and incorporated and pour them over the meatballs.
5. Set to cook on high for 2-3 hours or set to cook on low for 8 hours.

Keto Pot Roast

Calories: 307 Carbs: 1g Fat: 13g Protein: 10g
Servings: 4-5
Cooking: 4-5 hours

Ingredients:

- ✓ 1 tbsp./15ml olive oil
- ✓ ½ sliced onion
- ✓ ½ C. beef broth
- ✓ ½ C. /125ml mild pepper rings
- ✓ 1 pack of ranch dressing mix
- ✓ ½ C./125ml garlic butter
- ✓ 1-3 pounds of boneless beef roast

Preparation:

1. Pour the oil into a skillet and sear the beef on all sides. Place it into the crockpot.
2. Add all the other ingredients to the pot. Stir gently to combine.
3. Set to cook on low for 8-9 hours or set to cook on high for 4-5 hours.
4. Shred with forks and devour!

Beef Short Ribs with Creamy Mushroom Sauce

Calories: 365 Carbs: 1g Fat: 33g Protein: 13g
Servings: 8
Cooking: 6-8 hours

Ingredients:

- ✓ 1 tsp./4.93g pepper
- ✓ 1 tsp./4.93g salt
- ✓ 1 tsp./4.93g garlic powder
- ✓ 2 C./200g white mushrooms
- ✓ ½ C./120g beef broth
- ✓ 3 ounces/85.05g cream cheese
- ✓ 2 pounds/907.18g beef short ribs

Preparation:

1. In a skillet, brown the beef on all sides.
2. Mix together the pepper, salt, garlic powder, mushrooms, broth and cream cheese in your crockpot.
3. Place the ribs into the crockpot.
4. Set to cook on low for 6-8 hours. Stir every 1-2 hours during the cooking process.
5. Serve and Enjoy!

Crack Chicken

Calories: 275 Carbs: 4g Fat: 14g Protein: 11g
Servings: 8
Cooking: 6-8 hours

Ingredients:

- ✓ ½ pound bacon, cooked and crumbled
- ✓ 1 packet of ranch dressing mix
- ✓ 8 ounces cream cheese
- ✓ 1 pound boneless, skinless chicken breast

Preparation:

1. Place the dressing mix, cream cheese and chicken into the crockpot.
2. Set to cook on low for 6-8 hours or set to cook on high for 4 hours.
3. Shred with forks and mix in the bacon.
4. Serve & Enjoy!

Crispy and Juicy Crockpot Chicken Thighs

Calories: 577 Carbs: 1g Fat: 43g Protein: 44g
Servings: 4-6
Cooking: 6-7 hours

Ingredients:

- ✓ 6-8 bone-in, skin-on chicken thighs
- ✓ ½ tsp./2.5ml onion powder
- ✓ ½ tsp./2.5ml garlic powder
- ✓ ¾ tsp./5.75ml paprika
- ✓ 1 tsp./5ml salt

Preparation:

1. Mix the onion powder, garlic powder, salt and paprika together.
2. Coat the chicken thighs with seasoning mixture.
3. Place the chicken into your crockpot, skin side up.
4. Set to cook on low for 6-7 hours until tender.

Korean Spicy Pork

Calories: 189 Carbs: 7g Fat: 9g Protein: 15g
Servings: 4
Cooking: 2-3 hours

Ingredints:

Marinating and Cooking:

- ✓ ¼ C./62.5 ml water
- ✓ ¼ - 1 tsp./0.25 tsp. cayenne pepper
- ✓ 2 tbsp./30ml gochujang
- ✓ 2 packets Splenda
- ✓ 1 tbsp./15ml sesame oil
- ✓ 1 tbsp./15ml rice wine
- ✓ 1 tbsp./15ml coconut amino sauce
- ✓ 1 tbsp./15ml minced garlic
- ✓ 1 tbsp./15ml minced ginger
- ✓ 1 thinly sliced onion
- ✓ 1 pound/453.59g pork shoulder, sliced into cubes

Finishing:

- ✓ ¼ C./25g sliced green onions
- ✓ 1 tbsp./15ml sesame seeds
- ✓ 1 thinly sliced onion

Preparation:

1. Mix up all the marinade and ingredients in your crockpot. Let the mixture marinate for 60 minutes.
2. Set to cook on high for 2-3 hours.
3. Warm up a cast iron skillet. Add the pork cubes to the skillet along with the onion. Pour in ¼ - ½ cup of sauce.
4. Once the sauce has reduced down, and the onions are soft, sprinkle in the sesame seeds and green onions.
5. Serve!

Mushroom Lover's Pot Roast

Calories: 267 Carbs: 4g Fat: 16g Protein: 24g
Servings: 6
Cooking: 4 ½ - 5 hours

Ingredients:

- ✓ 1 – 1 ½ pounds cremini mushrooms
- ✓ 2-3 tsp./15ml olive oil
- ✓ ½ tsp./2.5ml pepper
- ✓ ¾ tsp./5.75ml salt
- ✓ 1 tsp./5ml onion powder
- ✓ 1-2 tbsp./10ml steak rub
- ✓ 3-4 pound chuck roast
- ✓ 2 mushroom stock cubes + ½ C. water

Preparation:

1. Pour the mushroom cubes and water into a bowl. Pop them into a microwave and heat for 60 seconds till dissolved. Stir well.
2. Trim the fat from the roast.
3. Mix up the steak rub, pepper, salt and onion powder together. Rub the mixture onto the roast.
4. Heat an iron skillet and brown the meat on all sides for 5-7 minutes. Place the meat into the crockpot.
5. Pour the mushroom stock mixture into a pan, cooking for 1-2 minutes. Scrape the bits from the bottom of the pan and pour them over the roast in the crockpot.
6. Set to cook on high for 3 hours.
7. Wash the mushrooms and slice them into thick pieces.
8. Place them over the roast after 3 hours and cook for another 45-60 minutes till the mushrooms are cooked through and the meat is nice and tender.
9. Scoop out the meat with the mushrooms. Strain the juices.
10. Slice the meat, place onto serving plates and top with cooked mushrooms and a spoonful of cooking juices.

Mexican Meatloaf

Calories: 246 Carbs: 6g Fat: 13g Protein: 26g
Servings: 8-12
Cooking: 5-6 hours

Ingredients:

- ✓ 1 C./250 ml shredded cheese of choice
- ✓ 19-ounce can enchilada sauce
- ✓ 1 celery stalk
- ✓ 1 carrot
- ✓ 1 red bell pepper
- ✓ 1 taco seasoning packet
- ✓ 1 onion
- ✓ 4.5-ounce can chopped green chilies
- ✓ 1/3 C./75 ml sour cream
- ✓ 1 egg
- ✓ 1 pound ground turkey
- ✓ 1 pound ground beef

Preparation:

1. In a big bowl, add both ground meats. Then add the taco seasoning, sour cream and egg
2. Trim the vegetables and dump them into a food processor. Process till smooth. Pour the veggie mixture into a bowl.
3. With your hands, mix up the ingredients till well combined. Shape the mixture into a log and place it into your crockpot.
4. Pour the enchilada sauce over the top.
5. Set to cook on low for 5-6 hours.
6. Sprinkle with cheese right before serving.

Beef and Broccoli

Calories: 564 Carbs: 6g Fat: 13g Protein: 26g
Servings: 3
Cooking: 2 hours

Ingredients:

- ✓ 2 tbsp./30ml Xantham Gum
- ✓ 5 minced garlic cloves
- ✓ ¼ C./60ml stevia
- ✓ ½ C. /125ml coconut amino sauce
- ✓ 1 C./250 ml beef stock
- ✓ 4 C./1l broccoli florets
- ✓ 1 ½ pounds beef flank steak, thinly sliced

Preparation:

1. Add the stevia, coconut amino sauce and beef stock to your crockpot. Stir to combine.
2. Then add the beef and coat it well with the sauce.
3. Set to cook on high for 2 hours.
4. Combine 2 tablespoons of cooking liquid with the Xantham Gum
5. Stir in the Xantham Gum mixture along with the garlic and broccoli.
6. Cook for another half an hour till the broccoli becomes tender.

Seafood Gumbo

Calories: 343 Carbs: 9g Fat: 12g Protein: 49g
Servings: 8
Cooking: 7 hours

Ingredients:

- ✓ 2 pounds deveined raw shrimp
- ✓ 1 ½ C./350ml bone broth
- ✓ 3 bay leaves
- ✓ ¼ C./60ml tomato paste
- ✓ 28 ounces diced tomatoes
- ✓ 4 diced celery ribs
- ✓ 2 diced bell peppers
- ✓ 2 diced yellow onions
- ✓ 3 tbsp./45ml Cajun seasoning
- ✓ 3 tbsp./45ml ghee
- ✓ 24 ounces sea bass fillets, cut into 2-inch chunks

Preparation:

1. Season the fillets with pepper and salt, sprinkling half of the Cajun seasoning.
2. Place the ghee into a skillet and saute the fillet chunks for 4 minutes. Add the remaining Cajun seasoning with celery, pepper and onions, sautéing for 2 minutes till fragrant.
3. Add the broth, bay leaves, tomato paste, diced tomatoes and cooked fish to the crockpot. Then mix in all the remaining ingredients, stirring well to incorporate.
4. Set to cook on low for 7 hours.

Salmon with Orange Ginger Sauce

Calories: 166 Carbs: 0g Fat: 8g Protein: 23g
Servings: 4
Cooking: 2 ½ hours

Ingredients:

- ✓ 2 tbsp./30ml no-sugar marmalade
- ✓ 1 – 1 ½ tsp./5.5ml pepper
- ✓ ½ - 1 tsp/5.5ml. salt
- ✓ 1 tsp./5ml minced garlic
- ✓ 2 tsp./10ml minced ginger
- ✓ 1 tbsp./15ml coconut amino sauce
- ✓ 1 pound/453.59g salmon

Preparation:

1. Place the salmon into a Ziploc bag.
2. Mix up all the other ingredients and pour them into the bag with the salmon. Marinate for 20-30 minutes.
3. Place the salmon along with the marinade sauce into your crockpot.
4. Set to cook on low for 2 hours.
5. Ensure the oven is preheated to broil.
6. Place the salmon into a piece of foil and broil for 3-4 minutes to crisp.

Protein Shrimp with Coconut Milk

Calories: 192 Carbs: 4g Fat: 12g Protein: 16g
Servings: 4
Cooking: 3-4 hours

Ingredients:

- ✓ ½ can unsweetened coconut milk
- ✓ 1 tsp./5ml garam masala
- ✓ ½ tsp./2.5ml cayenne pepper
- ✓ 1 tsp./5ml salt
- ✓ ½ tsp./2.5ml turmeric
- ✓ 1 tbsp./15ml minced garlic
- ✓ 1 tbsp./15ml minced ginger
- ✓ 1 pound/453.59g deveined and shelled shrimp

Preparation:

1. Mix all the ingredients together till well combined.
2. Pour the contents into your crockpot.
3. Set to cook on low for 7 hours or set to cook on high for 3 ½ - 4 hours.

Clam Chowder

Calories: 226 Carbs: 6g Fat: 18g Protein: 21g
Servings: 4
Cooking: 1 ½ hours

Ingredients:

- ✓ 3 cans whole clams
- ✓ 16 ounces bottled clam juice
- ✓ Pinch of cayenne pepper
- ✓ 1 tbsp./15ml whole, dried thyme
- ✓ 1 tbsp./15ml salt
- ✓ 4-5 C./1.5l peeled and diced celeriac root
- ✓ 1 ½ C./350ml diced onion
- ✓ 4 garlic cloves
- ✓ 2 pounds frozen cauliflower florets
- ✓ 1-quart chicken broth
- ✓ 8 ounces chopped bacon

Preparation:

1. Dice up the onions and peel and dice the celeriac root into ¼-inch pieces.
2. Sauté the bacon in a pan for 5-7 minutes till crispy. Place on a paper towel to drain.
3. Pour the cauliflower florets and broth into the crockpot.
4. Set to cook on high for 1 hour. Remove and pour into a blender along with the garlic. Blend until smooth and set to the side.
5. Add the onion and celeriac root to the crockpot. Then add the cayenne pepper, clam juice, pepper, thyme and salt. Mix well. Set to cook on high for 1 hour.
6. Add the cooked bacon and cauliflower puree. Stir everything well to incorporate thoroughly.
7. Pour the clams into a sieve and rinse them well.
8. Roughly chop the clams and mix them into chowder.
9. Adjust the seasonings as you see fit and enjoy!

Shrimp Fajitas

Calories: 308 Carbs: 5g Fat: 18g Protein: 27g
Servings: 4
Cooking: 5- 6 ½ hours

Ingredients:

- ✓ 1 tsp./5ml salt
- ✓ ½ tsp./2.5ml paprika
- ✓ 1 tsp./5ml chili powder
- ✓ 1 packet taco seasoning
- ✓ ½ C./125ml chicken broth
- ✓ 1 pound deveined and peeled raw shrimp
- ✓ 1 sliced onion
- ✓ 1 quartered tomato
- ✓ 2 sliced red peppers
- ✓ 2 sliced green peppers

Preparation:

1. Pour all the ingredients minus the shrimp into your crock pot. Set to cook on low for 5-6 hours.
2. Add the shrimp, mixing gently.
3. Cook on high for 30-45 minutes.
4. Serve!

Garlic Shrimp

Calories: 277 Carbs: 2g Fat: 9g Protein: 14g
Servings: 6-8
Cooking: 30 minutes

Ingredients:

- ✓ 1 tbsp./15ml parsley
- ✓ 2 pounds peeled and deveined large shrimp
- ✓ ¼ tsp./1.25ml crushed red pepper flakes
- ✓ ¼ tsp. /1.25ml pepper
- ✓ 1 tsp./5ml salt
- ✓ 1 tsp./5ml smoked paprika
- ✓ 6 thinly sliced garlic cloves
- ✓ ¾ C./175ml extra-virgin olive oil

Preparation:

1. Mix the red pepper flakes, pepper, salt, paprika, garlic and oil together in your crockpot. Set to cook on high for half an hour.
2. Add the shrimp, mixing well. Cook on high for 10 minutes. Stir and cook for an additional 10 minutes till the shrimp turns opaque in color.
3. Place the shrimp into a serving bowl
4. Pour some sauce over and garnish with parsley.
5. Enjoy!

Lemon Pepper Salmon

Calories: 165 Carbs: 1g Fat: 8g Protein: 13g
Servings: 3-4
Cooking: 1-2 hours

Ingredients:

- ✓ 1 carrot
- ✓ 1 red bell pepper
- ✓ 1 zucchini
- ✓ ½ thinly sliced lemon
- ✓ ½ tsp./2.5ml pepper
- ✓ ¼ tsp./1.25ml salt
- ✓ 3 tsp./15ml ghee
- ✓ 1 pound salmon skin-on fillet
- ✓ Few springs of basil, tarragon, dill, and parsley
- ✓ ¾ C./175ml water

Preparation:

1. Place the water and herbs into your crockpot. Place the salmon over the herbs, skin side down.
2. Drizzle the fillet with ghee and season with pepper and salt. Cover with lemon slices.
3. Set to cook on high for 1-2 hours.
4. While the salmon cooks, julienne cut your veggies.
5. Add the veggies to your crockpot and cook for another hour on high.
6. Serve the salmon with the lemon slices and sliced veggies.

Tilapia with Roasted Pepper Sauce

Calories: 251 Carbs: 2g Fat: 18g Protein: 11g
Servings: 3-4
Cooking: 1 ½ hours

Ingredients:

- ✓ ½ C./125ml grated parmesan cheese
- ✓ ¾ C./175 ml heavy cream
- ✓ 6 ounces pureed roasted peppers
- ✓ 6 ounces chopped roasted peppers
- ✓ 2 chopped garlic cloves
- ✓ 1 diced onion
- ✓ 3 tbsp./45ml butter
- ✓ 1 pound tilapia fillets

Preparation:

1. Add 2 tablespoons of butter to a skillet. Warm up and add the tilapia fillets, cooking for 3-4 minutes per side till thoroughly cooked.
2. Season the fillets with pepper and salt. Set to the side.
3. To the same skillet, add the remaining butter along with the diced onion. Sauté for 5 minutes.
4. Add the garlic to the onion along with the pureed and chopped roasted peppers, cooking for 5 minutes.
5. Pour in the parmesan cheese and heavy cream. Turn off the heat, stir and adjust the seasoning if needed.
6. Add everything to the crockpot and cook on high for 1 hour.
7. Garnish with parsley and more parmesan cheese.

Seafood Cioppino

Calories: 167 Carbs: 1g Fat: 19g Protein: 12g
Servings: 3-4
Cooking: 7 hours

Ingredients:

- ✓ ½ C./125ml chopped parsley
- ✓ 8 ounces lump crab meat
- ✓ 2 6.5-ounce cans minced clams in clam juice
- ✓ 1 pound raw shrimp
- ✓ 1 pound haddock fillets
- ✓ ½ tsp./2.5ml salt
- ✓ 2 bay leaves
- ✓ 2 tsp./10ml Italian seasoning
- ✓ 2 tbsp./30ml olive oil
- ✓ 2 tsp./10ml red wine vinegar
- ✓ 6 minced garlic cloves
- ✓ ½ C./125ml dry white wine
- ✓ 3 tbsp./45ml tomato paste
- ✓ 8 ounces clam juice
- ✓ 2 chopped celery stalks
- ✓ 1 diced yellow onion
- ✓ 28-ounce can diced tomatoes

Preparation:

1. Mix the salt, bay leaves, Italian seasoning, olive oil, vinegar, garlic, white wine, tomato paste, clam juice, celery, onions and tomatoes in your crockpot.
2. Set to cook on low for 6 hours.
3. Mix in the crab meat, clams, shrimp and haddock. Cook for another 45 minutes till the shrimp is pink and the haddock flakes with a fork easily.
4. Discard the bay leaves.
5. Ladle into serving bowls and devour!

Creamy Tomato Seafood Bisque

Calories: 345 Carbs: 3g Fat: 15g Protein: 10g
Servings: 3-4
Cooking: 45 minutes – 1 hour

Ingredients:

- ✓ 3 pounds seafood of choice (I like using bay scallops and shrimp)
- ✓ 2 tsp./10ml sherry
- ✓ 8 ounces cream cheese
- ✓ 29-ounce can diced tomatoes
- ✓ 6 C./2l chicken broth
- ✓ 2 tbsp./30ml honeyville almond flour
- ✓ 2 tsp./10ml oregano
- ✓ 1 bay leaf
- ✓ 1 minced garlic clove
- ✓ 2 chopped celery stalks
- ✓ 1 peeled and chopped carrot
- ✓ 1 chopped onion
- ✓ 5 tbsp./60ml butter

Preparation:

1. Add the butter, veggies and bay leaf to your crockpot. Cook on high for half an hour.
2. Add the flour, stir for a few minutes and add the broth, oregano and tomatoes. Cook for another half an hour.
3. Add the cream cheese and sherry, allowing the cheese to melt. Cook for 10 minutes.
4. Discard the bay leaf. With an immersion blender, puree the mixture until smooth.
5. Add the scallops and shrimp. Cook for 20-30 minutes until piping hot.
6. Garnish with parsley and season with pepper and salt before serving.

Spinach and Artichoke Casserole

Calories: 141 Carbs: 7g Fat: 9g Protein: 10g
Servings: 10
Cooking: 4-6 hours

Ingredients:

- ✓ 1 tbsp./15ml baking powder
- ✓ ¾ C./175ml honeyville almond flour
- ✓ ½ tsp./2.5ml pepper
- ✓ 1 tsp./5ml salt
- ✓ 3 minced garlic cloves
- ✓ 1 C./250 ml grated parmesan cheese
- ✓ 6 ounces chopped artichoke hearts
- ✓ 5 ounces chopped spinach
- ✓ ¾ C./175ml unsweetened almond milk
- ✓ 8 eggs

Preparation:

1. Grease the inside of your crockpot.
2. Whisk ½ of parmesan cheese, pepper, salt, garlic, artichoke hearts, spinach, eggs and almond milk together.
3. Add the baking powder and flour, combining well.
4. Spread them into the crockpot. Sprinkle with the remaining parmesan cheese.
5. Set to cook on high for 2-3 hours or set to cook on low for 4-6 hours.
6. Serve!

Noodle Bowl with Creamy Curry Sauce

Calories: 110 Carbs: 1g Fat: 9g Protein: 7g
Servings: 4
Cooking: 1-2 hours

Ingredients:

- ✓ 2 handfuls of mixed greens
- ✓ Chopped cilantro
- ✓ 1 diced red bell pepper
- ✓ ½ head chopped cauliflower
- ✓ 2 chopped carrots
- ✓ 1 pack of Shirataki Noodles

Curry Sauce:

- ✓ ¼ tsp./1.25ml ginger
- ✓ ½ tsp./2.5mlpepper
- ✓ 1 tsp./5ml cumin
- ✓ 1 tsp./5ml turmeric
- ✓ 1 ½ tsp./5.5ml coriander
- ✓ 2 tsp./10ml curry powder
- ✓ 2 tbsp./30ml apple cider vinegar
- ✓ ¼ C./60ml water
- ✓ 2 tbsp./30ml avocado oil
- ✓ ¼ C./60ml avocado oil mayo

Preparation:

1. Add all the ingredients, minus the curry sauce ingredients, to your crockpot. Set to cook on high for 1-2 hours.
2. In the meantime, add all the curry sauce ingredients to a blender. Puree until smooth.
3. Pour over the veggie and noodle mixture. Stir well to coat.
4. Serve!

Vegetarian Cream of Mushroom Soup

Calories: 281 Carbs: 3g Fat: 16g Protein: 11g
Servings: 2
Cooking: 1 ¾ hours

Ingredients:

- ✓ ½ diced yellow onion
- ✓ 1 ½ C. diced white mushrooms
- ✓ ½ tsp. extra-virgin olive oil
- ✓ ¼ tsp. sea salt
- ✓ 1 tsp. onion powder
- ✓ 1 2/3 C. unsweetened almond milk
- ✓ 2 C. cauliflower florets

Preparation:

1. Add the cauliflower, pepper, salt, onion powder and milk to the crockpot. Stir and set to cook on high for 1 hour.
2. Sauté the onion and mushrooms in olive oil for 8 minutes.
3. Allow the cauliflower mixture to cool off and add it to a blender. Blend until smooth. Then blend in the mushroom mixture.
4. Pour this back into the crockpot and heat for 30 minutes.
5. Serve & Enjoy!

Kelp Noodles with Avocado Pesto

Calories: 321 Carbs: 1g Fat: 32g Protein: 2g
Servings: 2
Cooking: 1 ½ hours

Ingredients:

Pesto:

- ✓ 1-2 garlic cloves
- ✓ 1 tsp./5ml salt
- ✓ ¼ C./60ml basil
- ✓ 1 C./250 ml baby spinach leaves
- ✓ ½ C./125ml extra-virgin olive oil
- ✓ 1 avocado
- ✓ 1 package of kelp noodles

Preparation:

1. Add the kelp noodles to your crockpot with just enough water to cover them. Cook them on high for 45-60 minutes.
2. In the meantime, combine the pesto ingredients in a blender, blending till smooth and incorporated.
3. Stir in the pesto and heat the noodle mixture for 10 minutes.
4. Serve!

Vegan Bibimbap

Calories: 119 Carbs: 0g Fat: 18g Protein: 8g
Servings: 4
Cooking: 45 minutes

Ingredients:

- ✓ 2 tbsp./30ml sesame seeds
- ✓ Liquid sweetener
- ✓ 1 tsp./5ml sesame oil
- ✓ 1 tbsp./15ml coconut amino sauce
- ✓ 2 tbsp./30ml rice vinegar
- ✓ 2 tbsp./30ml sriracha sauce
- ✓ 10 ounces riced cauliflower
- ✓ ½ cucumber, sliced into strips
- ✓ 1 grated carrot
- ✓ 4-5 broccoli florets
- ✓ 1 sliced red bell pepper
- ✓ 7 ounces tempeh, sliced into squares
- ✓ 2 tbsp./30ml rice vinegar

Preparation:

1. In a bowl, combine the tempeh squares with 1 tbsp. coconut amino sauce and 2 tbsp. vinegar. Set them aside to soak. Slice the veggies.
2. Add the carrot, broccoli and peppers to your crockpot. Cook on high for 30 minutes.
3. Add the cauliflower rice to the pot, cook for 5 minutes.
4. Add the sweetener, oil, coconut amino sauce, vinegar and sriracha to your crockpot. Don't hesitate to add a bit of water if you find the mixture too thick.
5. Serve & Enjoy!

Mushroom Risotto

Calories: 438 Carbs: 5g Fat: 17g Protein: 12g
Servings: 4
Cooking: 3-4 hours

Ingredients:

- ✓ 1/3 C./75 ml grated parmesan cheese
- ✓ 4 tbsp./60ml butter
- ✓ 3 tbsp./45ml chopped chives
- ✓ ¼ C./60ml vegetable broth
- ✓ 2 diced shallots
- ✓ 1 pound sliced white mushrooms
- ✓ 1 pound sliced Portabello mushrooms
- ✓ 3 tbsp./45ml coconut oil
- ✓ 4 ½ C./1.5l riced cauliflower

Preparation:

1. Heat up the oil and sauté the mushrooms for 3 minutes till soft. Discard the liquid and set to the side.
2. Add the oil to a skillet and sauté the shallots for 60 seconds.
3. Add all the ingredients to your crockpot. Stir well.
4. Set to cook on high for 3 hours.
5. Serve topped with parmesan cheese.

Twice Baked Spaghetti Squash

Calories: 230 Carbs: 4g Fat: 17g Protein: 12g
Servings: 4
Cooking: 6 hours

Ingredients:

- ✓ 4 slices Provolone cheese
- ✓ ¼ tsp./1.25ml pepper
- ✓ ¼ tsp./1.25ml salt
- ✓ 1 tsp./5ml oregano
- ✓ 2 minced garlic cloves
- ✓ ½ C./125ml grated parmesan cheese
- ✓ 2 tbsp./30ml butter
- ✓ 2 small spaghetti squash

Preparation:

1. Slice the squash(es) in half and scoop out the innards. Place them into your crockpot.
2. Set to cook on high for 4 hours.
3. Take the squash innards and mix them with parmesan cheese and butter. Then mix in the pepper, salt, garlic and oregano.
4. Add the squash innards mixture to the middle of the cooked squash halves.
5. Cook on high for another 1-2 hours till the middles are bubbly.

Zucchini Pasta

Calories: 181 Carbs: 6g Fat: 13g Protein: 5g
Servings: 4
Cooking: 1-2 hours

Ingredients:

- ✓ ½ tsp./2.5ml crushed red pepper flakes
- ✓ ½ C./125ml basil
- ✓ ¼ C./60ml extra-virgin olive oil
- ✓ 4 minced garlic cloves
- ✓ 1 sliced red onion
- ✓ 1 pint halved cherry tomatoes
- ✓ 2 pounds spiralized zucchini

Preparation:

1. Sauté the onion and garlic for 3 minutes till fragrant in olive oil.
2. Add the zucchini noodles to the crockpot and season with pepper and salt. Cover and cook on high for 1 hour.
3. Add tomatoes, basil, onion, garlic and red pepper. Cook for another 20 minutes.
4. Add the parmesan cheese to your crockpot. Mix thoroughly and cook for 10 minutes.

Keto Crack Slaw

Calories: 360 Carbs: 5g Fat: 33g Protein: 7g
Servings: 2
Cooking: 1 ¾ hours

Ingredients:

- ✓ 2 garlic cloves
- ✓ 1 tbsp./15ml sesame oil
- ✓ 2 tbsp./30ml tamari
- ✓ 1 tsp./5ml vinegar
- ✓ 1 tsp./5ml chili paste
- ✓ ½ C./125ml chopped macadamia nuts
- ✓ 4 C./1l shredded cabbage

Preparation:

1. Toss the cabbage in the chili paste, sesame oil, vinegar and tamari. Add them to your crockpot.
2. Add the minced garlic and mix well.
3. Set to cook on high for 1 ½ hours.
4. Stir in the macadamia nuts. Cook for 5 minutes more.
5. Garnish with sesame seeds.

Stuffed Eggplant

Calories: 180 Carbs: 2g Fat: 13g Protein: 9g
Servings: 6
Cooking: 1 ½ hours

Ingredients:

- ✓ 1 tbsp./15ml tomato paste
- ✓ 1 tsp./5ml cumin
- ✓ 1 tsp./5ml stevia
- ✓ 4 chopped tomatoes
- ✓ 1 seeded and chopped green bell pepper
- ✓ 3 tbsp./45ml chopped parsley
- ✓ 4 minced garlic cloves
- ✓ 2 chopped red onions
- ✓ 4 tbsp./60ml olive oil
- ✓ 6 eggplants

Preparation:

1. Remove the eggplant skins with a vegetable peeler. Slice the eggplants lengthwise and sprinkle with salt. Allow to sit for half an hour to sweat.
2. Place the eggplants into your crockpot. Cook on high for 20 minutes.
3. Sauté the onions in a skillet using olive oil until softened. Add the garlic and bell pepper, sautéing for 2 minutes.
4. Add the mixture to the eggplants inside the crockpot. Cook for 20 minutes on high.
5. Season with pepper and salt and add the parsley, tomato paste, cumin, stevia and tomato.
6. Cook for another 10 minutes, stir well and serve!

Cheesy Bacon Cauliflower

Calories: 278 Carbs: 2g Fat: 17g Protein: 6g
Servings: 6
Cooking: 3-4 hour

Ingredients:

- ✓ 3 ounces bacon crumbles
- ✓ 1 ½ C./350ml grated mozzarella cheese
- ✓ 2 C./500ml unsweetened almond milk
- ✓ ¼ tsp./1.25ml pepper
- ✓ ½ tsp./2.5ml salt
- ✓ ¼ C./60ml honeyville almond flour (keto friendly)
- ✓ ¼ C./60ml butter
- ✓ 2 pounds cauliflower florets

Preparation:

1. Place the cauliflower florets into your crockpot.
2. In a pan, melt the butter and mix in the pepper, salt and flour.
3. Add the milk and simmer until the mixture begins to bubble.
4. Add the cheese and stir until its smooth. Pour it over the cauliflower and combine.
5. Set to cook on low for 3-4 hours.
6. Mix in the bacon. Season as desired.

Keto Green Beans

Calories: 101 Carbs: 1g Fat: 11g Protein: 4g
Servings: 6
Cooking: 4-5 hours

Ingredients

- ✓ 14.4-ounce can chicken broth
- ✓ 2 pounds fresh green beans (ketogenic friendly beans)
- ✓ 1 tbsp./15ml butter
- ✓ 2 minced garlic cloves
- ✓ 1 diced yellow onion

Preparation:

1. Sauté the garlic and onion together for 7-10 minutes. Add them to your crockpot.
2. Add the green beans and chicken broth to the crockpot.
3. Set to cook on low for 4-5 hours.
4. Season as needed. Enjoy!

Keto Stuffing

Calories: 256 Carbs: 2g Fat: 21g Protein: 9g
Servings: 10
Cooking: 3-4 hours

Ingredients:

- ✓ 2 eggs
- ✓ 3-4 C./1l chicken broth
- ✓ Fresh herbs of choice
- ✓ ¼ C./60ml parsley
- ✓ 12 C. cubed tempeh
- ✓ 2 C./500ml chopped celery
- ✓ 2 diced onions
- ✓ 2 tsp./10ml poultry seasoning
- ✓ ½ tsp./2.5ml salt
- ✓ ½ tsp./2.5ml pepper
- ✓ 1 C./250 ml butter

Preparation:

1. Heat the butter in a pan and add the pepper, salt and poultry seasoning. Stir well.
2. Add the onions and celery to your pan, sautéing till soft. Allow to cool completely.
3. In a bowl, add tempeh cubes with the cooled celery and onions. Mix in the parsley and chicken broth. Then add in the eggs.
4. Cover and chill overnight for the tempeh to marinate.
5. Grease your crockpot well. Add the stuffing mixture to the pot.
6. Set to cook on low for 3-4 hours.
7. Serve!

Pepper Jack Cauliflower

Calories: 272 Carbs: 6g Fat: 21g Protein: 11g
Servings: 6
Cooking: 1 hour

Ingredients:

- ✓ 6 slices cooked and crumbled bacon
- ✓ 4 ounces shredded pepper jack cheese
- ✓ ½ tsp./2.5ml pepper
- ✓ 1 tsp./5ml salt
- ✓ 2 tbsp./30ml butter
- ✓ ¼ C. /60mlwhipping cream
- ✓ 4 ounces cream cheese
- ✓ 1 head cauliflower, sliced into 1-inch florets

Preparation:

1. Grease your crockpot.
2. Add all your ingredients, except for the pepper jack cheese, to your crockpot. Stir well.
3. Set to cook on low for 3 hours.
4. Stir in the pepper jack cheese and cook for another 30-60 minutes until the cauliflower is nice and tender.
5. Stir in the bacon crumbles and devour!

Parmesan and Chive Mashed Cauliflower

Calories: 190 Carbs: 2g Fat: 18g Protein: 7g
Servings: 4-6
Cooking: 2-3 hours

Ingredients:

- ✓ ¼ C./60ml chopped chives
- ✓ ¼ C./60ml grated parmesan cheese
- ✓ 2 C./500ml chicken broth
- ✓ 2 small cauliflower heads, cored and sliced into florets

Preparation:

1. Add all the ingredients to your crockpot, stir well.
2. Set to cook on high for 2-3 hours.
3. Season with pepper and salt and sprinkle with additional parmesan.
4. Serve!

Celery Root and Cauliflower Puree

Calories: 167 Carbs: 1g Fat: 8g Protein: 4g
Servings: 6-8
Cooking: 5 hours

Ingredients:

- ✓ 3 tbsp./45ml butter
- ✓ ½ tsp./2.5ml salt
- ✓ 1 head cauliflower sliced into florets
- ✓ 1 celery root sliced into ½-inch cubes

Preparation:

1. Add all the ingredients to your crockpot and combine well.
2. Set to cook on high for 5 hours till the cauliflower and celery root are tender.
3. With an immersion blender, slightly blend the mixture until its smooth.

Coconut Lime Cauliflower Rice

Calories: 215 Carbs: 2g Fat: 14g Protein: 8g
Servings: 9
Cooking: 4-5 hours

Ingredients:

- ✓ 2 tsp./10ml lime zest
- ✓ 1 tbsp./15ml chopped cilantro
- ✓ 2 tbsp./30ml water
- ✓ 2 tbsp./30ml coconut oil
- ✓ 3 tbsp./45ml unsweetened almond milk
- ✓ 2 C./500ml chopped cauliflower

Preparation:

1. Combine all the ingredients in your crockpot.
2. Set to cook on high for 4-5 hours.

Cauliflower Hummus

Calories: 97 Carbs: 0g Fat: 12g Protein: 5g
Servings: 10
Cooking: 4 hours

Ingredients:

- ✓ ¾ tsp./.75ml salt
- ✓ 3 tbsp./45ml extra-virgin olive oil
- ✓ 2 crushed garlic cloves
- ✓ 3 tbsp./45ml lemon juice
- ✓ 1 ½ tbsp./25ml tahini paste
- ✓ 3 garlic cloves
- ✓ ½ tsp./2.5ml salt
- ✓ 2 tbsp./30ml avocado oil
- ✓ 2 tbsp./30ml water
- ✓ 3 C. /750ml cauliflower florets

Preparation:

1. Add all the ingredients to your crockpot.
2. Set to cook on high for 4 hours.
3. With an immersion blender, blend the mixture until creamy and smooth.

Bacon and Gouda Cauliflower Mash

Calories: 147 Carbs: 2g Fat: 10g Protein: 7g
Servings: 4-6
Cooking: 4 hours

Ingredients:

- ✓ 1/3 C./75 ml shredded smoked gouda cheese
- ✓ 4 slices cooked bacon
- ✓ ¼ tsp./1.25ml garlic powder
- ✓ ¼ tsp./1.25ml pepper
- ✓ ½ tsp./2.5ml salt
- ✓ 2 tbsp./30ml butter
- ✓ 3 tbsp./45ml. heavy cream
- ✓ 4 C./1l cauliflower florets

Preparation:

1. Add all the ingredients to your crockpot, combining well.
2. Set to cook on high for 4 hours.
3. With a potato masher, gently mash the mixture till just slightly chunky.

Parmesan Zucchini Tots

Calories: 175 Carbs: 1g Fat: 19g Protein: 11g
Servings: 10
Cooking: 3-4 hours

Ingredients:

- ✓ 1 egg
- ✓ ½ C./125ml shredded parmesan cheese
- ✓ ½ tbsp./7.5ml Italian seasoning
- ✓ 1 ½ C./350ml shredded zucchini

Preparation:

1. Add the shredded zucchini to your crockpot.
2. Combine with the remaining ingredients, mixing thoroughly.
3. Set to cook on high for 3-4 hours till the zucchini is tender.
4. Remove the mixture and shape it into small "tot" shapes.
5. Line a sheet with parchment paper and bake for 15-20 minutes at 400 degrees till crispy.

Blueberry Lemon Custard Cake

Calories: 375 Carbs: 4g Fat: 27g Protein: 14g
Servings: 8-9
Cooking: 3 hours

Ingredients:

- ✓ ½ C./125ml fresh blueberries
- ✓ 2 C./500ml light cream
- ✓ ½ tsp./2.5ml salt
- ✓ ½ C. /125ml sweetener of choice
- ✓ 1 tsp./5ml lemon stevia
- ✓ 1/3 C./75 ml lemon juice
- ✓ 2 tsp./10ml lemon zest
- ✓ ½ C./125ml honeyville almond flour
- ✓ 6 separated eggs

Preparation:

1. Into a stand mixer, add the egg whites. Whip till soft peaks are created. Set to the side.
2. Whisk the yolks with the remaining ingredients minus the blueberries. Fold in the egg whites.
3. Grease the crockpot and pour in the batter. Sprinkle with blueberries.
4. Set to cook on low for 3 hours.
5. Allow to cook for at least 1 hour and then chill for at least 2 hours or overnight.
6. Serve!

Keto Chocolate Cake

Calories: 357 Carbs: 5g Fat: 26g Protein: 13g
Servings: 6-7
Cooking: 2 ½ hours

Ingredients:

- ✓ 1/3 C./75ml sugar-free chocolate chips
- ✓ ¾ tsp./1.75ml vanilla extract
- ✓ 2/3 C./150ml unsweetened almond milk
- ✓ 6 tbsp./90ml melted butter
- ✓ 3 eggs
- ✓ ¼ tsp./1.25ml salt
- ✓ 1 ½ tsp./25ml baking powder
- ✓ 3 tbsp./45ml whey protein powder
- ✓ ½ C. /125ml cocoa powder
- ✓ ½ C./125ml Swerve
- ✓ 1 C./250 ml + 2 tbsp. honeyville almond flour

Preparation:

1. Grease your crockpot.
2. Mix the salt, baking powder, protein powder, cocoa powder, sweetener and flour together.
3. Mix in the vanilla, almond milk, eggs and butter. Fold in the chocolate chips.
4. Pour them into your crockpot.
5. Set to cook on low for 2 ½ hours.
6. Let them cool and then slice them into pieces.
7. Serve & Enjoy!

Lemon Crock Pot Cake

Calories: 310 Carbs: 4g Fat: 29g Protein: 8g
Servings: 8
Cooking: 2-3 hours

Ingredients:

- ✓ 2 eggs
- ✓ Zest of 2 lemons
- ✓ 2 tbsp./30ml lemon juice
- ✓ ½ C./125ml whipping cream
- ✓ ½ C./125ml melted butter
- ✓ ½ tsp./2.5ml xanthan gum
- ✓ 2 tsp./10ml baking powder
- ✓ 3 tbsp./45ml swerve sweetener
- ✓ ½ C./125ml coconut flour
- ✓ 1 ½ C./350ml honeyville almond flour

Topping:

- ✓ 2 tbsp./30ml lemon juice
- ✓ 2 tbsp./30ml melted butter
- ✓ ½ C./125ml boiling water
- ✓ 3 tbsp./45ml swerve sweetener

Preparation:

1. Combine the xanthan gum, baking powder, sweetener and flour together.
2. Whisk the egg, lemon juice and zest, whipping cream and butter together.
3. Combine the wet and dry mixtures together till well incorporated. Pour them into a greased crockpot.
4. For the topping, combine all the topping ingredients till incorporated and spread them over the top of the cake mixture.
5. Set to cook on high for 2-3 hours.
6. Serve warm with whipped cream and fresh fruit!

Chocolate Molten Lava Cake

Calories: 418 Carbs: 4g Fat: 27g Protein: 8g
Servings: 12
Cooking: 3 hours

Ingredients:

- ✓ 2 C./5ooml hot water
- ✓ 4 ounces sugar-free chocolate chips
- ✓ ½ tsp./2.5ml vanilla liquid stevia
- ✓ 1 tsp./5ml vanilla extract
- ✓ 3 egg yolks
- ✓ 3 whole eggs
- ✓ ½ C./125ml melted and cooled butter
- ✓ 1 tsp./5ml baking powder
- ✓ ½ tsp./2.5ml salt
- ✓ 5 tbsp./60ml unsweetened cocoa powder
- ✓ ½ C./125ml honeyville almond flour
- ✓ 1 ½ C./350ml swerve sweetener

Preparation:

1. Grease your crockpot liberally.
2. Whisk the baking powder, salt, 3 tbsp. cocoa powder, flour and 1 ¼ C. swerve together.
3. Stir the liquid stevia, vanilla, yolks, eggs and melted butter together.
4. Combine the wet and dry mixture till well incorporated. Pour them into the crockpot.
5. Top with chocolate chips. Mix in the remaining swerve and cocoa powder.
6. Set to cook on low for 3 hours.
7. Serve & Enjoy!

Pumpkin Custard

Calories: 419 Carbs: 4g Fat: 16g Protein: 19g
Servings: 8-10
Cooking: 2-3 hours

Ingredients:

- ✓ 4 tbsp./60ml butter
- ✓ 1/8 tsp./25ml salt
- ✓ 1 tsp./5ml pumpkin pie spice
- ✓ ½ C./125ml honeyville almond flour
- ✓ 1 tsp./5ml vanilla extract
- ✓ 1 C./250 ml pumpkin puree
- ✓ ½ C./125ml granulated stevia
- ✓ 4 eggs

Preparation:

1. Grease the inside of your crockpot.
2. Beat the eggs until smooth. Then beat in the sweetener, gradually. Add the vanilla and pumpkin puree until blended well.
3. Then mix in the pumpkin pie spice, salt and almond flour. Blend as you add in the butter. Pour into the crockpot.
4. Place a paper towel over the opening of the pot before closing it.
5. Set to cook on low for 2 – 2 ¾ hours.
6. Serve warm with whipped cream and a dash of nutmeg!

Keto Crock Pot Cheesecake

Calories: 301 Carbs: 2g Fat: 31g Protein: 23g
Servings: 12
Cooking: 2-3 hours

Ingredients:

- ✓ ½ tbsp./7.5ml vanilla extract
- ✓ 1 C./250 ml stevia
- ✓ 3 eggs
- ✓ 3 8-ounce packages of cream cheese

Preparation:

1. Allow the cream cheese to warm up to room temperature.
2. Cream the cheese with the stevia until blended. Then add the eggs, one at a time, beating after each addition. Blend in the vanilla.
3. Grease a pan or bowl well and add cream cheese mixture to it.
4. Add 2-3 cups of water into the bottom of the crockpot.
5. Add the pan to pot. Set to cook on high for 2 – 2 ½ hours.

Blackberry Chocolate Chip Cake

Calories: 289 Carbs: 5g Fat: 19g Protein: 9g
Servings: 10-12
Cooking: 3 hours

Ingredients:

- ✓ 1/3 C./75 ml dark chocolate chips (sugar-free)
- ✓ 1 C./250 ml blackberries
- ✓ ½ C./125ml heavy cream
- ✓ ¼ C./60ml melted butter
- ✓ ¼ C./60ml melted coconut oil
- ✓ 4 eggs
- ✓ ¼ tsp./1.25ml salt
- ✓ 2 tsp./10ml baking soda
- ✓ ¼ C./125ml chocolate whey protein powder
- ✓ ½ swerve sweetener
- ✓ 1 C./250 ml unsweetened shredded coconut
- ✓ 2 C./500ml honeyville almond flour

Preparation:

1. Grease the inside of your crockpot with butter.
2. Mix all the dry ingredients together. Then add in all the wet ingredients, blending well to ensure adequate incorporation.
3. Pour batter into the prepared crockpot.
4. Set to cook on low for 3 hours.
5. Serve topped with more blackberries!

Crockpot Keto Apple Cider

Calories: 178 Carbs: 1g Fat: 8g Protein: 5g
Servings: 12-15
Cooking: 3 hours

Ingredients:

- ✓ 7 C. water
- ✓ ¼ C./60ml maple syrup
- ✓ ¼ C./60ml stevia
- ✓ 1 tsp./5ml allspice berries
- ✓ 2 tsp./10ml whole cloves
- ✓ 3 cinnamon sticks
- ✓ 1 sliced orange
- ✓ 6 apples of choice, cored and sliced

Preparation:

1. Pour all the ingredients into your crockpot and pour water over everything.
2. Set to cook on high for 3 hours.
3. Discard the orange slices and cinnamon sticks.
4. With an immersion blender, blend the mixture until smooth.
5. Cook for another hour on high.
6. Strain the mixture through a cheesecloth.
7. Add back to the pot to keep warm.
8. Serve & Enjoy!

Keto Zesty Lemon Cake

Calories: 250 Carbs: 2g Fat: 16g Protein: 11g
Servings: 10
Cooking: 6-8 hours

Ingredients:

- ✓ Zest of 1 lemon
- ✓ 4 eggs
- ✓ ½ C./125ml unsweetened almond milk
- ✓ 1/3 C./75 ml butter
- ✓ 1 tsp./5ml baking soda
- ✓ 2 tsp./10ml cream of tartar
- ✓ 2 tsp./10ml vanilla extract
- ✓ ½ C./125mlswerve sweetener
- ✓ ¼ C./60ml plain egg protein powder
- ✓ ¼ C./60ml coconut flour
- ✓ 2 C./500ml honeyville almond flour

Filling:

- ✓ 1 C./250 ml low-carb lemon curd
- ✓ 1 tsp./5ml vanilla extract
- ✓ 1 C./250 ml coconut cream

Glaze:

- ✓ 2 tbsp./30ml swerve sweetener
- ✓ Zest of 1 lemon
- ✓ 1 tbsp./15ml lemon juice
- ✓ 2 tbsp./30ml coconut oil
- ✓ ½ C./125ml coconut butter

Preparation:

1. Combine the almond milk and butter together. Then mix in the vanilla, eggs and lemon zest.
2. Combine all the dry ingredients together. Then combine the wet and dry mixtures, combining well.
3. Line a springform pan with parchment paper and pour batter into it.
4. Place the pan into the crockpot and cook on low for 2 hours.
5. Take out and place in a fridge for 4-6 hours to chill.
6. To prepare the filling, combine all the ingredients together until smooth. Do the same with the glaze.
7. Cut the cake in half. Fill one part of the cake with filling, lay the other half over the top and then drizzle with glaze. Tip with additional lemon zest.

Lemon Cheesecake Mousse

Calories: 156 Carbs: 1g Fat: 17g Protein: 14g
Servings: 5-7
Cooking: 30 minutes

Ingredients:

- ✓ 1/8 tsp./.25ml salt
- ✓ ½ - 1 tsp./5ml lemon liquid stevia
- ✓ 1 C./250 ml heavy cream
- ✓ ¼ C./125ml lemon juice
- ✓ 8 ounces cream cheese

Preparation:

1. In a mixer, add the lemon juice and cream cheese. Blend until smooth.
2. Add the heavy cream along with the remaining ingredients, blending till well incorporated.
3. Adjust the sweetener if needed.
4. Pour the mix into your crockpot. Set to cook on low for 30 minutes.
5. Pour into serving glasses and chill for 5 hours or overnight.
6. Serve topped with lemon zest.

Cooking Notes

Cooking Notes

Cooking Notes

Cooking Notes

Cooking Notes

Made in the USA
San Bernardino, CA
03 October 2018